GET IT UP!

Revealing the Simple,
Surprising
Lifestyle that Causes…

Migraines,
Alzheimer's,
Stroke,
Glaucoma,
Sleep Apnea,
Impotence…
and More!

GET IT UP!

Revealing the Simple,
Surprising
Lifestyle that Causes…

Migraines,
Alzheimer's,
Stroke,
Glaucoma,
Sleep Apnea,
Impotence…
and More!

Sydney Ross Singer
Soma Grismaijer

ISCD
PRESS

Published by:

ISCD PRESS
P.O. Box 1880
Pahoa, Hawaii 96778
U.S.A.

ISCD PRESS is the publication branch of the Institute for the Study of Culturogenic Disease, a program of the Good Shepherd Foundation, Inc., a non-profit research and education foundation.

Library of Congress Catalogue Card Number (LCCN): 00-190973

ISBN: 1-930858-00-0

Other Books by Singer and Grismaijer:

Get It Off! Understanding the Cause of Breast Pain, Cysts, and Cancer, Illustrated with A Little Breast Play (ISCD Press, HI 2000) ISBN 1-930858-01-9

Get It Out! Eliminating the Cause of Diverticulitis, Kidney Stones, Bladder Infections, Cervical Dysplasia, PMS, Menopausal Discomfort, Prostate Enlargement...and More! (ISCD Press, HI 2001) ISBN 1-930858-02-7

The Doctor Is Out! If you've been told you have high blood pressure, low thyroid, or diabetes, you may be a victim of one of the mist common medical scams of our time. (ISCD Press, HI 2001) ISBN 1-930858-04-3

Dressed To Kill: The Link Between Breast Cancer and Bras (Avery, NY 1995) ISBN 0-89529-664-0

Printed in Canada

10 9 8 7 6 5 4 3 2

To Camela, with love.

Acknowledgements

We would like to thank Monday Magazine and journalist/ author William Thomas, the Times Colonist newspaper, the Victoria News, Terry Spence at CFAX radio station, and Karen Ledger of the Canadian Health Education And Research (CHEAR) Foundation for their support of the Migraine Relief Project. We also would like to express our appreciation to the participants in the Project, who were willing to open their minds to new ideas and to alter their lifestyles to better their health. And a special thanks goes to Dorrie Murphy for her research assistance.

In addition, we wish to thank Daryl and Anthea Archer at Fairburn Farm, John Park, Peggy Cady, and Brian and Sylwia Mackie for their friendship and encouragement. They showed us what good Canadian hospitality is all about and made us feel at home.

For critical review of the manuscript for this book, we wish to thank Mark Wyse, M.D., who is one of the leading family medicine practitioners in Phoenix, Arizona; Dr. Darrell Stoddard, founder of the Pain Research Institute in Provo, Utah; Ralph Reed, Ph.D., Biochemist/toxicologist at Oregon State University, who also volunteered many hours of research support; and journalist Julie Jansen who offered valuable support and input. A special thanks goes to Alan Hargens, Ph.D., Professor of Orthopedics, University of California, and Senior Research Physiologist, Gravitational Research Branch, NASA Ames Research Center, for his encouragement and critical review.

We wish to thank Danny and Burna O'Toole for their friendship, support, and assistance. And we wish to express our appreciation to veteran actor John Phillip Law for his continuing support and generosity.

Finally, we wish to thank the Divine Source that has empowered us with this lifesaving information. We are grateful and humbled by the responsibility we feel this information has bestowed upon us for the sake of humanity.

Contents

Dear Reader

We are proud to present to you the most ambitious work ever achieved by the Singer and Grismaijer research team. As you read these pages, you will witness the explosion of a myth about migraines, Alzheimer's, glaucoma, sleep apnea, impotence, and other conditions that plague our culture at this time in history. The myth is that these conditions are disconnected problems, each with its own mystery cause, and that the individuals wishing to avoid or recover from them need to have drugs or surgery. It is a myth that has generated "associations" and "foundations" for each problem, many of which are funded, at least in part, by drug industry money; it has created a massive cadre of researchers making a career studying these problems; it has cost billions of dollars from taxpayers to subsidize these research efforts, and to pay again for the product of that research, which are drugs that only treat, never cure, and have dangerous side effects; and it has kept millions of people suffering needlessly from diseases that their very own lifestyles have created.

The key to our health and disease is our lifestyles. It is due to lifestyle that some cultures have "senior" citizens living into their 20's, other cultures into their 40's, others into their 80's, and others into their 100's. Why the difference? We are all human. All other things being equal, shouldn't all human beings live to a similar age and have similar health? Aren't we all cut from the same biological "cloth"?

The reason for the difference is due to the way that "cloth" is fashioned. Each culture fashions the attitudes and behaviors of its citizens, and these determine the health of those citizens.

When filth was in fashion in western cultures 200 years ago, for example, epidemic diseases kept the population and life expectancy low. Once the fashion for cleanliness in body, water and food supply, and general urban sanitation became popular, the life expectancy rose as the disease rate fell. The cause of the disease and death was not the bacteria in the filth or the genetic make-up of the people. It was the cultural assumption that being clean was unimportant, if not unhealthful. Once the culture cleaned up its act, the health of its citizens improved.

Before this change in attitude had become culturally acceptable, some of the filthiest people of all were doctors. Occupationally, doctors are exposed to infectious diseases. Unaware at the time of the need to wash their hands, doctors inadvertently served as the spreaders of disease. They even knew about bacteria back then. They just refused to believe that such small things could harm a big human being. It took decades, and the self-sacrificial determination of people like Ignaz Philipp Simelweis, Oliver Wendell Holmes, and Louis Pasteur, to sway medicine from its dirty course. Cultural patterns die hard.

The moral of this story is that medicine is also a product of the culture, equally bound as any other profession or occupation to the same set of cultural assumptions and practices that bind, and blind, all people. This means that medical doctors and researchers are like the blind leading the blind when it comes to identifying culture-caused, or culturogenic, disease. Medical "experts" wear the same type of clothing as everyone else; they use the same soaps, shampoos, and cleansers as everyone else; they eat like everyone else; they drive the same types of vehicles, use the same phones, televisions, computers, and radios, read the same newspapers, see the same movies, and sleep in the same kinds of beds as everyone else. If any one of these behaviors causes disease, they will suffer from it like everyone else. And since cultural patterns are taken for granted and are rarely questioned, they will be ignorant of the cause of the disease like everyone else.

This means that you cannot turn to medicine for answers to the cultural causes of disease, since medicine is also a product of the culture. Believing that you can is another myth that this book will explode. In addition, medicine is a disease treatment industry. It profits from the treatment of disease. The more people are sick, the more money is made by the medical industry.

Entire medical sub-industries have developed around brain, sleep, and sexual problems, with billions of dollars spent on research, drugs, and hospitalization. There are thousands of new medical articles written yearly about these problems, with no solution in sight but new drug treatments to sell.

Imagine discovering the simple lifestyle cause and solution to those problems. You could finally prevent these problems, instead of having to treat them. And you could save millions of people pain, suffering, and death by explaining what they need to *stop* doing that is making them sick in the first place. It would be a dream come true. Except, that is, for the army of people who make a living treating those problems.

When a disease generates industries that profit from its existence, it will be difficult to eradicate the disease without resistance from those industries. Nobody likes to see others sick; but nobody likes to lose his or her job, either.

This is the essential dilemma for eliminating culture caused diseases. Disease can be profitable for some industries. This creates a conflict of interest between those who suffer, and those who make a living on that suffering.

This is not a personal issue. People profiting from disease are not evil. Most of these people are dedicated professionals trying to alleviate suffering. But they are working within a system that profits from disease. So long as industries profit from disease, they will be invested in those diseases continuing.

These, then, are the two powerful factors that resist the prevention and cure of culture caused disease: we wear blinders that keep us from honestly and clearly examining our own behaviors and attitudes; and we have entrusted our health to a disease treatment industry. The result is a culture that inadvertently causes sickness, and then becomes invested in that sickness continuing.

You are just one little person out of a billion people participating in this culture. When many people and industries profit from a damaging lifestyle that you are practicing, your suffering caused by that lifestyle may be a price that the culture is willing for *you* to pay. Only, these days there are too many little people having to pay that price. That's why there is so much money now going into medicine.

This means that your culture is making you sick. Frankly, we care more about health than about the culture. We are willing to do something "different", if it means being healthier. And we have proven on ourselves personally, and on others through our applied medical anthropology research, that these "different" behaviors really make a difference.

Your health care is really a lifestyle issue. In this report, we will explain to you what we believe is the lifestyle that causes brain disease, and more. It is a simple solution to an extremely complex, convoluted, and almost unintelligible field of medicine. But if health were a complex issue, then no living creature would ever survive.

This report will hopefully start a revolutionary new trend in *self-care*. We will tell you how to *PREVENT* disease and *LIVE HEALTHFULLY* by understanding how your lifestyle affects your health.

We are not here to sell you drugs.

We are here to tell you truths.

Of course, you can serve some people truth on a silver platter, and they only take the platter. And sometimes it is easier to sell falsehoods than to give away truths.

So be it. But if we don't tell you the truth, who will?

Once you finish this book you will be empowered with information that can extend your life and improve its quality. It will all be up to you. Will you escape the cultural trap that has ensnared people for centuries? Will you join the elite brotherhood of humankind that, each generation, has risen above the cultural ignorance and biases that bind the mind and destroy the body and spirit?

We hope so.

S.R.S. & S.G.,
May, 2000

Introduction

This is more than a report on the cause and cure of migraines. It is the story of the discovery of a lifestyle problem that leads to more diseases than you could imagine. In fact, we never dreamed that our first steps into the complicated world of migraine research would lead us to such diseases as Alzheimer's, Parkinson's, and even impotence. As we write this report, we are expanding our understanding of the impact of this discovery on health and disease. As we continue to research these implications of our new theory, you can help us by performing your own SELF STUDY, as we will explain later on. When you finish reading what follows, we expect that you will be as shocked as we are that this information is not commonplace. And we expect that those participating in a SELF STUDY will experience a renaissance of health they never imagined as possible.

We will start our report at the beginning – with our quest for the cause of migraines. Migraines can destroy lives. There are few things worse than facing life as a migraineur. It means living in constant fear – fear of the pain; fear of the trigger; fear of what it is doing to their lives and loved ones; and fear of what else might happen to their brains. Migraines isolate people from others as they suffer in their own private hell.

Amazingly, it may be a hell of their own making!

We have discovered that migraines are preventable and curable. It only takes a simple lifestyle change that, to our astonishment, has never before been considered in research on migraines. And we have proven the validity of our theory with research results from our Migraine Relief Project.

As applied medical anthropologists, we use the fields of biochemistry, anthropology, and medicine to research the causes of disease. We believe that health is our inheritance from nature. We have evolved to live, not to suffer. The problem is that our lifestyles get in the way. Our goal is to discover those lifestyles that can lead to particular diseases. And we believe that we have found the lifestyle that may cause migraines, Alzheimer's disease, glaucoma, Parkinson's disease, stroke, Sudden Infant Death Syndrome (SIDS), sleep apnea, seizures, impotence, and more.

We have come to our discovery by piecing together the many fragments of the migraine puzzle. Then we added a crucial piece that somehow had eluded research into migraines for the past 100 years. This crucial piece is not a chemical, or a nerve, or a gene. While it has been ignored in migraine research, it is a critical aspect of all head conditions. And its neglect has foiled more than migraine research, confounding virtually all brain studies.

How can something so fundamental be ignored? As a culture, we do not analyze that which is ever present. The exception is far more interesting than the rule. Of course, this means that we frequently ignore the obvious, such as the effect of gravity on our bodies and brains.

We have reasoned, using established medical facts, that gravity and reduced brain circulation are the keys to migraines. It has to do with the way we sleep. Gravity affects you differently when you are asleep, and horizontal, than it does when you are awake, and vertical.

When standing, gravity reduces the blood pressure delivering blood to the brain, and aids the drainage of blood from the brain. When lying down, this effect of gravity is lost, and fluid pressure builds in the head and brain. In the morning, after anywhere from 6-12 hours of sleep, during which time the brain has had limited circulation and high pressure, the signs of fluid accumulation are apparent in puffy eyes, stuffy sinuses, and a groggy, congested brain.

We will show how this gravity effect may possibly be the mechanism for creating migraines. We will describe in detail this revolutionary new theory, exploring its universal application to many health conditions. And we will show how we successfully tested our theory, presenting our research from the Migraine Relief Project.

We will also suggest how the reader can perform a free and safe SELF STUDY to see whether the lifestyle change we are recommending can alleviate headaches, improve memory, return libido, and, in general, revitalize the brain and body. Finally, we will provide references to other medical studies that directly or indirectly support our theory. And we will try to explain why 100 years of research has failed to come up with the causes of these problems, producing little more than confusion, fatalism, and expensive drugs for treatment.

We hope that the discovery we have made will provide relief to millions whom, as you will see, may be needlessly suffering from migraines, Alzheimer's disease, stroke, and other head conditions. We also encourage further research into this sleep theory we are about to present, which may prove to be the Rosetta stone of brain research.

1

Brain Pain

We were not born to suffer. But it's hard telling that to someone with migraines.

Camela, Soma's 20-year-old daughter, knew suffering. Throughout the past ten years that I have known her, she has been a physically attractive but shy girl. In fact, her shyness was one of her most characteristic features, and it seemed to keep her from engaging in the normal activities of childhood and young adulthood. She frequently complained about headaches, slept ten or more hours daily, and sometimes had a groggy, puffy look to her face, especially her left side. She slowly developed a sense of apathy towards the world, and a deep feeling that there was something wrong with her, which prevented her from engaging in normal activities. Nobody, however, knew that she suffered from migraines, not even herself. She knew that she suffered, of course. But no one suspected that it was migraines. Camela, herself, secretly thought that she had a brain tumor, which would explain the pain she frequently felt on the left side of her head.

It was unusual for Camela to talk about herself or to analyze her feelings, which kept her problem her own personal nightmare. But on one particular rainy day, with all of us stuck inside the house forced to deal with one another's attitudes and behaviors, her apathy had gotten the best of me, and I began to harass her for not doing more with her life. It was then that she admitted to seeing strange things, like flashes of light. Sometimes everything went blank. These frightening visual disturbances, combined with the constant tension in her head and recurrent severe headaches, convinced Camela that she had a brain disease, and that she would never be able to participate in life as a normal person.

This had been the first time that Camela shared with anyone her deep felt fears and realities regarding her brain. It had taken her years to face her problem directly. I immediately suspected that she had been seeing auras, a feature of classic migraines, and went to my medical books to read what I could about migraines. As I shared the information with Camela I could see her facial expression change. It was as though a huge burden had been lifted from her poor soul. No, she did not have a brain tumor. It was only migraines.

The Migraineur

Only migraines!? As I read further, I discovered that virtually nothing is known about the cause of this condition. People who suffer from migraines are told that they may suffer for life, and are even given a label all their own, the "migraineur". It is a common condition, with some estimates suggesting that it affects 15-25% of the public. It is considered a vascular headache, meaning that it is somehow connected to the blood supply to the brain. The headaches are recurrent, are typically on one side of the head, and can last for several hours or days. Associated with the headache can be a sense of malaise, nausea, vomiting, and sensitivity to light. Sometimes certain neurological problems precede the headache, such as bright flashing lights; burning, tingling, or numbness in the hand or around the mouth; muscular weakness on one side of the body; sensory defects on one side of the body; and speaking difficulty. The side of the body affected is opposite the side with the headache, which reflects the medical fact that the left side of the brain controls the right side of the body, and vice versa. If the migraine has these early neurological signs prior to the onset of the headache, then it is called a classic migraine. Otherwise, if you go straight to the headache, it is called a common migraine. Most migraines are the common type. The disorder usually begins in childhood, affects women more than men, and can run in families.

Tension Headaches

Almost everyone has a headache every now and then. Most headaches are stress related, caused by tight muscles in the jaw, neck, scalp, or brow. Some headaches are caused by eyestrain or dental problems. Tension headaches are often confused with migraines, and can be constant for days, weeks or months. In fact, many people with migraines also suffer from tension headaches. This should be no surprise. If you had to go through life with the constant prospect of a severe, disabling, killer headache hitting you at any time, it would be enough to give you a tension headache. A tension headache, however, may respond to massage. We can personally attest to relieving our own headaches by gently feeling the head for tight muscles and massaging them until they are no longer firm and painful, at which time the headache disappears. Spinal adjustment of the neck vertebrae may help relieve headaches, too.

Migraine Triggers

Migraines are different. They are not muscular headaches, but vascular ones, which means that they relate to the brain's blood supply. The arteries in the neck dilate, increasing the amount of blood coursing through the brain. If you press on these arteries during an attack it can temporarily relieve the pain, only to have it return with increased severity when you let go. What sets off the headache? With a tension headache, it could be the stress of your lifestyle. With a migraine, it could be anything. These so-called triggers of migraines can literally be any food, smell, sound, visual stimulus, or thought. It is as though any stimulation of the brain can elicit a migraine attack.

As I explained all this to Camela her relief in not having a brain tumor turned to confusion. What was she to do? It's great to get a diagnosis of your problem so you can know what is wrong with you. But what do you do with a problem that is not going away? Of course, the standard medical answer is drugs. Lots of them. All of your life. Side effects and all.

What a terrible thing to tell someone. "Sorry, dear, but you are going to have severe headaches all your life and you need to take these dangerous, expensive drugs just to get by. They won't cure you, since you are incurable. But they will make it easier to live through your attacks." I couldn't tell Camela that. So much research has gone into the mechanism of migraines. Why does nobody understand the cause of this condition? Could it be that migraines are not the problem that people think they are?

Dealing With Symptoms

Knowing the cause of a problem is essential to treating it. Otherwise, you can only treat symptoms. However, if you treat symptoms you may be interfering with the natural processes by which the body is trying to deal with the problem.

For example, let's assume you are a physician and you are asked to treat a feverish patient who has some generalized infection. If you do not know the cause of the infection, you cannot properly treat it. If it is bacterial, for example, you may want to use an antibiotic. But which bacterium is causing the infection is a critical issue, since antibiotics are specific for certain bacteria. So you cannot know which antibiotic to use without knowing the identity of the bacterium. And if it is a virus causing the infection, the use of antibiotics is useless, since they do not affect viruses. You may want to take a blood sample to determine the offensive microorganism so you can better prescribe a treatment. However, this will take time, and the patient still has an uncomfortable but not life-threatening fever of, let's say, 102 degrees Fahrenheit. In the absence of knowing the cause, do you treat the symptoms? Should you, for example, treat the patient for the fever, giving drugs such as aspirin or ibuprofen to lower it?

According to standard medical practice, in the absence of being able to treat the cause, treat the symptoms. Headache, stuffy nose, fever, nausea are all signs and symptoms of disease. Look for a cause, but treat the symptoms in the meantime, which will make the patient feel more comfortable. That is the medical approach to patient care.

But is this the wise approach?

Looking at Lifestyle

We must disclose our professional bias. As applied medical anthropologists, our emphasis is on the lifestyle causes of disease, not the treatment. We believe that it is better to prevent disease than to treat it once it occurs. We have training in biochemistry, anthropology and medicine and use these to understand human health and disease in a different way than that typically promoted in medicine. To us, the human body has been designed to function properly, whether as an outcome of millions of years of evolution, or as the product of a powerful, all knowing Creator. The problem is that people get in the way of that proper functioning as a result of culturally defined behaviors and attitudes. The World Health Organization tells us that about 70%-80% of our deaths are due to lifestyle.[1] The message is simple: the way we are living goes against the way our bodies are supposed to work. And it's killing us.

Lifestyle, of course, is a cultural issue. Our culture tells us how to live. It gives us thoughts and dreams. It clothes us and feeds us. It makes the world meaningful for us. All of our values are cultural products. All of our aspirations stem from cultural norms and values. We are conditioned by our culture in the womb, as we sense the sounds and flow of the world outside. We even die as our culture tells us, and are put in the final resting-place our culture has deemed fitting. It is our culture that gives us identity. And we cannot understand ourselves without understanding our culture.

Nature versus Culture

Unfortunately, there is a conflict between our nature and our culture. Our nature is our internal design meant to allow us to live healthfully. Our culture, however, is forever trying to alter this nature, as the fashions of the time dictate. Of course, nature provides a great degree of latitude in its design, to allow for a broad range of environmental realities in which the organism may have to live. But people do like to push the limits. After all, you don't know where your limits are until you try to exceed them.

In the desire to become the master of his own fate, man has identified nature as the fundamental enemy to conquer. Why accept limits imposed by nature? The mind of man can elevate us above those limits. Or so the reasoning goes. As a result, genetic engineering is in vogue, with the desire to be re-designers of the natural world. Of course, there are still natural laws on Earth that we cannot get around, such as the law of gravity. That which we cannot change is usually ignored.

Nature as the Enemy

This cultural antagonism towards nature manifests in the field of medicine as a disregard for the natural healing processes of the body. Modern medicine cannot consider nature the hero. It treats it as the enemy. Getting back to our example of the infection with a fever, the doctor will see the fever as part of the problem, not as part of the body's solution to the problem. Fortunately, many people, including some doctors, now realize that the purpose of a fever is to enhance the function of the immune system, which operates better under fever conditions. White blood cells, which are the "foot soldiers" of the immune system, are more active at higher body temperatures. This mechanism shows that the body is not helpless when it deals with assaults to its integrity and health. Our minds may not understand the processes, but our bodies instinctively know what to do.

In summary, our view of health and disease is that we are typically healthy if we live according to nature's design. We get sick when our culture gets in the way. The predominant medical view is that we need our culture and its medicines to keep the ravages of nature from disabling and killing us.

Signs and Symptoms

The medical bias against nature is reflected in the very language it uses, and forces all of us to use, in the description of disease. When you have a fever, for example, it is considered a "symptom" of a disease. What is a symptom? It is a manifestation of an illness experienced by an individual. In distinction to this is the word "sign" which is the manifestation of an illness as objectively measured by a doctor. A disease, then, has signs and symptoms. The only difference is that symptoms are subjective and signs are objective. Both, however, are considered manifestations of an illness or disease.

But a fever is not a manifestation of a disease, despite what medicine says. It is a manifestation of the body's ability to fight the disease. It is a process by which the body tries to rid itself of the disease. If you think of fever as a symptom of disease, then you will see it as an evil, hurtful thing, which must be fought. If you think of fever as a manifestation of the body's healing power, then you will see it as a wonderful thing, which must be supported.

This illustrates the power of words in framing the thoughts of man, and the ultimate power of culture in the creation of our realities. Our culture gives us those words with which to think and conceptualize the world. When we define all bodily processes associated with a disease as a manifestation of that disease, then we see the symptoms as something to fight. Interestingly, we cannot speak of "healthy symptoms" or "good signs", since the terms "symptom" and "sign" imply illness, not a healthful response to an illness. A "healthy symptom" is an oxymoron. There is no single word to express a normal, healthy bodily response to disease, such as a fever. To modern medicine, everything that goes on when you are sick is unhealthy and must be stopped. Otherwise, how could a doctor justify treating "symptoms" in the absence of knowing the cause of a disease?

The Cultural Cause of Disease

What happens, we believe, is that people are getting sick due to something that they have done, most likely something that their culture has conditioned them to do, which is contradictory to the natural requirements for health, and they get sick. Their bodies then develop defense strategies and maneuvers to manage the illness, which are good responses to a bad thing. And until the bad thing that started the problem in the first place is stopped, the problem will not go away. Meanwhile, modern medicine, ignorant of the cause of the problem, attempts to stop the mechanisms by which the body is trying to heal. The result is that the problem never goes away, and even gets worse, since the natural defense mechanisms have been defeated. Guess who loses.

Could this be the case with migraines? The cause is unknown, which means treatment is merely a shot in the dark, which may or may not make matters worse. Could a migraine be a natural, healthy mechanism for trying to deal with a deeper, unnatural problem? Some researchers have suggested that migraines may serve a survival function.[2] In other words, are migraines the fire or the smoke alarm?

I had never before thought much about migraines apart from my medical school training. But insight often comes when you are outside the problem. Camela was so relieved that she didn't have a brain tumor that the prospect of another headache seemed less frightening. She agreed to be one of our research subjects as we further explored the issue. But we had no leads to go on. Clearly, everyone has been looking in the wrong direction, or there would have been an answer by now as to the true cause of migraines. We needed to find a new direction. All the migraine research was so confused.[3]

However, confusion is a state of mind, not a state of reality. We decided to think about migraines with a fresh, unbiased perspective. After all, truth cannot enter a closed door.

Later that night, as I stumbled out of bed, I discovered our first big clue.

2

The Brain in a Nutshell

With these new thoughts I retired for the night, only to awaken a few hours later hearing a strange sound. As I arose from my bed to investigate, I began to feel dizzy. My stomach felt nauseated and I held onto the wall to keep myself up, for I sensed the possibility that I might faint. My heart pounded and I instinctively lowered my head, which made it feel better. After a few moments, the problem stopped. I had experienced a phenomenon called orthostatic hypotension. It is a common phenomenon, not indicative of any disease, and attributable to blood pressure changes in the head upon rising from a flat position. This was an important clue in understanding migraines. However, we must first review some basic brain anatomy and physiology to fully understand its significance.

There is much that could be said about the brain. In medical school we had to take several courses in neurophysiology, examining and identifying various parts of the brain. Besides the gross anatomy, there is the histology of the brain, with the microscopic examination of the various brain cell types. This information can be found in any good textbook on the brain. Be cautioned, however, that it is easy to get lost in the trees of this forest. We will try to provide you with the information you will need to understand the arguments that follow.

The Brain's Need for Nutrients

The brain is perhaps the most complicated organ in our bodies. Its function is to integrate our internal world and coordinate its relationship to the external world. Our senses are special outcroppings of our brain. The brain not only receives stimuli from the external world, but also packages them into perceptions and conceptions and elicits a response to them. The brain is the seat for our thoughts and emotions. It also puts out hormones, which affect other organs of the body.

Due to its importance, the brain commands a great deal of the body's blood supply and nutrients. The brain and spinal cord, which is the tail of the brain communicating messages between itself and the rest of the body, possess the highest resting metabolic rate of any large organ of the body, meaning that it is more active in its resting state than any other organ. It consumes 20% of the body's resting oxygen requirement. Its primary food is glucose, the sugar commonly found in our blood. The brain has practically no reserve of oxygen and very little reserve of sugar, making it extremely vulnerable to a reduction in blood supply. Yet, it is remarkably capable of caring for itself, as you would expect of such an important organ. It possesses internal autoregulatory processes that allow it to support normal, or nearly normal, function despite blood flow reductions down to 40% of normal. Below this threshold physiological dysfunction occurs, and only a small additional decline in blood supply causes death of brain cells.

Circulation of the Brain

The blood supply to the brain is through 4 major arteries. If you feel your throat on either side of your Adam's apple you will feel the pulse of the common carotid artery. This main artery branches into the internal and external carotid arteries. The external branch feeds blood to the face and scalp and all the structures outside the skull bone. The internal carotids pass into the skull to feed the brain. Two other arteries pass into the skull through the neck bones, called the vertebral arteries. You cannot feel their pulse because they are protected by the vertebrae of the neck. The two internal carotid arteries and the two vertebral arteries meet in the brain much in the same way as roadways do when coming to a traffic circle. The circle where they meet is called the Circle of Willis, and its significance is that the blockage of any one of the arteries can be compensated for by the other arteries, ensuring that the brain receives an adequate blood supply. These arteries branch further as they go to their targeted brain area to supply it with oxygen and nutrients.

The arteries, of course, get progressively smaller as they approach the area they are to serve, turning into arterioles. Brain arterioles are different from arterioles outside the brain. They are less elastic and have less muscle inside their walls. However, there are muscles surrounding special resistance arterioles, which can adjust their internal diameter in response to the metabolic requirements of the brain and to changes in systemic blood pressure. This means that these arterioles open wider to allow more blood to pass when the part of the brain that they are serving needs more oxygen and sugar. This happens when part of the brain begins to work more. Other parts of the brain that are not being used as much can have relatively less blood flow, so arterioles to those parts are more constricted, allowing less blood to flow through. Also, if the blood pressure to the brain is too high, the arterioles may close down to increase the resistance and reduce blood flow, in order to prevent the brain from getting too pressurized. Conversely, if the blood pressure is too low, the arterioles may open wider to allow more blood to enter the brain. This internal ability of the brain to alter its circulation is termed autoregulation, which means the brain does it by itself. Autoregulation balances the needs of different functional parts of the brain for blood, taking into consideration the blood pressure of the body, which provides the blood, and the metabolic needs of the brain tissue. This autoregulation allows the brain to operate with blood pressure as low as 60 mm Hg (millimeters of mercury) and as high as 160 mm

Hg without trouble. Normal blood pressure is between 80mm Hg and 120 mm Hg.

The Blood-Brain Barrier

One other difference of the brain blood supply is the so-called blood-brain barrier. The arterioles get even smaller and become capillaries which feed the brain tissue. Fluid oozes out of the capillaries, carrying with it oxygen and sugar. Unlike other capillaries, however, this oozing is extremely selective. Other capillaries of the body have spaces between the cells lining their insides, which can allow proteins and other large molecules to pass through into the surrounding tissue spaces. The brain, however, is extremely selective in what it allows through due to tighter cellular junctions in the capillary lining.

Nutrients and oxygen pass through the capillary blood into the brain tissue space, and waste, such as carbon dioxide, is returned to the blood by diffusion from the tissue spaces. The capillaries then come together to form small veins, called venules, which converge into larger venules. These eventually empty into one of various venous sinuses, which are large blood collection vessels. The main one is called the superior sagittal sinus, and is located on the top of the brain, running from the front to the back. Other blood collection sinuses exist, and these sinuses merge. To get the blood out of the head and back to the heart, veins lead down from these sinuses. The principal veins are the right and left internal jugular veins.

Cerebral Spinal Fluid

That's only part of the story. Besides bringing blood to the brain for nourishment and oxygenation, the cerebral arteries bring blood to the center of the brain for the creation of cerebral spinal fluid. Within the center of the brain are several caverns, called ventricles. There are four ventricles in total. These are the right and left lateral ventricles, the third ventricle, and the fourth ventricle. Narrow tube-like passageways connect these ventricles. There are specialized capillary beds within the ventricles that ooze a fluid similar to lymph fluid secreted by the capillaries of the rest of the body, only with less protein in the fluid due to the tighter cellular junctions of the blood-brain barrier. (Lymph fluid is the straw colored liquid that you find in a blister. This fluid bathes our body's tissues, just as cerebral spinal fluid bathes the brain's tissue.) The cerebral spinal fluid fills up the ventricles, and provides a fluid cushion for the inside of the brain. Out of the fourth ventricle there are holes through which cerebral spinal fluid gets to the outside surface of the brain and around the spinal cord, to keep the brain moist and cushioned from blows.

Obviously, too much fluid in the ventricles would be a bad thing, putting pressure on the brain structures next to the ventricles and pressurizing the brain. This is what happens with intracranial (within the brain) hypertension (elevated pressure). More on that later.

Orthostatic Hypotension Explained

There is one further detail that you need to understand the phenomenon I experienced when rising from bed and getting dizzy. The carotid arteries in the neck have pressure receptors within them to detect blood pressure. If the pressure is high the brain risks getting too much fluid pressure, which can blow a blood vessel and cause bleeding in the brain, which is called a cerebral vascular accident, or stroke. In addition to the brain's intrinsic autoregulation for pressure control, the carotid arteries can provide extra support by giving negative feedback to the heart to reduce its pumping rate and force, lowering blood pressure.

Now, let's examine the phenomenon I experienced. When I first lay down in bed my blood pressure was normal for a *standing* position. But as my head touched the pillow, my carotid arteries immediately sensed a rise in pressure, and so did my brain. Why did the pressure increase in my head and neck? It was due to gravity, or, more accurately, to the negation of gravity.

When standing, blood must pump up, against gravity, to supply the brain, so the pressure has to be high. When you lower your head, blood is pumped directly into the head without the resistance of gravity, raising the pressure within the brain. The brain does not want too much pressure, so the carotid arteries and brain react to the increased pressure that occurs when first lying down by lowering the heart's rate and pumping force, and by constricting the resistance arterioles within the brain. This is why heart rate and blood pressure are lower when we sleep. It keeps us from having a stroke.

Why did I get dizzy when I arose? Since I had been down for some time, my blood pressure had been low. A sudden rising to the upright (orthostatic) position brought gravity back into the equation, without giving the heart enough warning time to pump harder in order to lift the blood up to my now vertical head. This momentarily caused excessively low blood pressure (hypotension), depriving my brain of sufficient blood and causing me to be dizzy, nauseated, and feeling faint. As my brain quickly responded, it signaled my heart to pound. My reflexive response of lowering my head helped supply my brain with more blood pressure while my heart tried to adjust. After a few moments, my blood pressure rose to the point where I felt normal again standing.

I stood there in the bedroom contemplating the significance of this experience. The key was gravity. Gravity is one of those natural laws that we tend to ignore. It is everywhere, making it so obvious a part of our lives that we easily overlook its presence. Yet, it is one of the main natural forces affecting pressure within the brain. Everything I have told you about the brain I had learned in medical school. But gravity was never mentioned. Its effect on the brain, however, is obvious and irrefutable. We live in a gravity field, and it affects us differently when we are horizontal than when we are vertical. An interesting theory began to develop in my mind. Could gravity be the key to migraines?

3

The Gravity of Migraines

Sleep is as mysterious to us as birth and death. We can only see it happening to others. Yet we spend anywhere from 25%-50% of our lifetimes doing it. And we need to sleep at certain intervals to keep healthy. It's clearly an important part of our lives.

It is therefore surprising how little time is spent by most people thinking about and managing this time in their lives. Perhaps it is because we do not experience our sleep. We only experience our dreams. In addition, our culture thinks of sleeping as a time to relax and let the worries and efforts of the day behind. It is a time to stop reflection, not start it. Consequently, we fail to ever fully reflect on sleep.

However, its effect on you will be apparent throughout the night and in the morning — the aches and pains, the stuffy sinuses and baggy eyes, and the groggy head. And, sometimes, the headache. Are these the required outcome of sleeping, or can we get through the night without having them to deal with in the morning?

The first thing to realize about sleep is that we do it lying down. Let's assume that a person sleeps 8 hours per night on the average. That means he will spend 16 hours awake. Let's assume, further, that he spends this 16 hours either standing or sitting, but not lying down. This means that while vertical for two thirds of the day, this person will have his heart above his feet and below his head. While sleeping for one third of the day, all of his body will be on the same horizontal plane.

The Effect of Gravity on the Brain

During the day, as this person stands, blood is pumped each second out of his heart and up, against gravity, to reach his head. At the same time gravity pulls blood down from the head back to the heart. Meanwhile, the legs are getting the benefit of both gravity and heart pumping to receive blood. However, the force of gravity resists the flow of blood from the legs back to the heart. This blood, having already lost most of its pressure from the heart, must weakly climb uphill. It achieves this remarkable defiance of gravity through the help of nearby contracting muscles, which squeeze the blood up successive segments of veins separated from one another by gated, one-way valves.

Yet, we are living organisms who fatigue, while gravity is an ever-present force. Gravity always wins in the end. So by the end of the day our brains feel drained. And when we look at our feet and ankles we may see swollen tissue, which represents the fluid that gravity has claimed over the day.

One benefit of sleep is that we get some time off from gravity. As this person lies down, blood pumped from the heart need no longer fight uphill to reach the head. Now, it liberally gushes in. In fact, its flow is so copious and powerful that the brain must reduce its intensity, lowering the pulse and blood pressure and closing down some of its resistance arterioles. And gravity no longer provides the pull that facilitates drainage of the brain's veins. So the result of lying down is increased intracranial, or inside of the head, pressure throughout the night as compared to during the day. Of course, the feet are enjoying their time decongesting, since gravity no longer keeps the blood accumulated there.

Vertical time, then, causes the brain to drain and the feet to swell. Horizontal time causes the feet to drain and the brain to swell.

Side Sleeping

However, we have not really gotten rid of gravity. We really can't, here on earth. Our bodies simply experience gravity differently when horizontal, which depends on our sleep posture. You can sleep on your side, on your stomach, or on your back. Each posture has different consequences. In fact, you can tell whether a person is a side sleeper and on which side he sleeps by simply looking at his face. His nose will be bent away from the side he predominantly sleeps on. Try it. It works. Faces are asymmetrical because some people smash their face into a pillow for one third to one half of their lives. As they age this effect becomes more marked, and you can even see the cheek on the same side become more stretched out and puffy than on the side of the face spared the daily compression. The facial skin, in general, will suffer from compression, developing wrinkles and other signs of pre-mature aging.

In addition to facial skin stretching, wrinkling, and reshaping, the sinuses and ear on the down side become congested. Hearing may even become impaired in the down ear relative to the up ear. Then there is the nose. The physical compression of the lower nostril into the pillow effectively closes off half of the nose. This makes breathing difficult, raising the blood carbon dioxide levels and lowering the oxygen levels.

One of the autoregulatory processes in the brain includes response to carbon dioxide levels. When these levels are high, the brain opens up its resistance arterioles to allow more blood to get through to flush out the carbon dioxide and replace it with oxygen. This means that reducing one's ability to breathe by closing off a nostril with the pillow can lead to changes in the brain. And these changes lead to further pressurizing of the brain in the horizontal state by further opening up the brain's arterioles.

Finally, one other effect of side sleeping is that it may lead to the impingement of the veins draining the brain. Many people sleep with their neck firmly nestled in a pillow. This reduces the ability for blood to drain from the brain, further adding to the pressurizing effect. Of course, the carotid artery can also become impinged, which would have the opposite effect, reducing blood delivered to the brain. But it takes a lot more pressure to impinge a high pressure, thick-walled artery than to impinge a low pressure, thin-walled vein. In either event, pressure on the neck when sleeping can interfere with brain circulation.

Sleeping position can effect more than the brain, altering circulation and causing compressions to various parts of the body, inside and out. In chapter 6 we will discuss more about sleep position and what we believe is the correct way to sleep. The point we wish to make at this time is that how we sleep clearly affects our physiology, leading to possible pressure changes in the brain.

Of course, this pressurizing of the brain is a good thing, up to a point. It compensates for the time we spend erect, when gravity drains the brain. But the process can get excessive. Just as the feet can swell, so can the brain.

Time Up versus Time Down

How long should it take for the brain to repressurize? Everyone would have their own answer to this question, and it would change daily depending on many variables. Clearly, however, the longer you lie down, the longer your head pressurizes, and the less time you have depressurizing in a vertical position. There are only 24 hours in a day. Those who sleep for 6 hours and are vertical for 18 have a 3:1 ratio of vertical to horizontal time. Those who sleep 12 hours daily have a 1:1 ratio, significantly different from the less somnolent individual. And both of these ratios may be appropriate for the individuals living them. We must each be our own standard, since we are each unique beings living unique lives. But you can

24

usually tell if people are mismatched with their sleep patterns by the way they look and feel when getting up.

If you are not down long enough, then you will feel fatigued. Your brain hasn't had enough time to recharge its pressure. If you had too much time down, then you might also feel fatigued, but will also have other signs of head pressurization, such as congested sinuses, and a puffy face and eyes. Your face will show the excess pressure in the head. If your face is swollen, then so is your brain.

Brain Edema

What is wrong with a congested brain? As with all congested tissue, swelling reduces the ability for oxygen and carbon dioxide to diffuse through the tissue, leading to pockets of stagnant liquid low in oxygen, which has already been consumed by metabolism, and high in carbon dioxide, one of the waste products of that metabolism. Nutrients, such as sugar, that have already been consumed by metabolism are also difficult to replace in stagnant tissue. This condition of excess fluid accumulation is called edema. It is a sad state in which cells are sitting in their own waste, starved of oxygen and nutrients, and it can ultimately lead to cell death and tissue destruction. But before that end arrives, there is a slow, progressive deterioration of tissue structure and function due to the chronic, or long-standing, congestion.

Edema is a problem for all tissues, but more so for the brain. First, there is a skull to consider. The brain cannot swell for long before the skull limits the expansion and the brain begins to compress itself. This can result in strange experiences, such as hallucinations, or tingling in the arms. Second, there is the fact that the brain is devoid of a lymphatic system. The lymphatic system consists of tiny, microscopic vessels that drain our body's tissues of fluid and debris. Edema is typically relieved by drainage of the tissue via the lymphatic system. Lacking it, the brain takes a much longer time ridding itself of the edema.

Once the brain becomes repressurized during its horizontal

time, excess pressurization would lead to brain edema. Ventricles within the brain might swell and impinge on surrounding brain tissue. The brain stem, the part of the brain responsible for our basic vital functions, such as breathing and heart rate, will try to intervene, telling the sleeping person whose skull it is in that it's time to get up. If the person listens to the message and arises, the brain can begin to again use gravity to drain its fluids and to resist the pressure of blood coming from the heart.

However, what happens if this "wake up call" is ignored? Our culture tells us to ignore it, especially if it comes in the middle of the night. "I have to go to work in the morning," we reason, "and I can't take a nap in the middle of the day. So I had better make myself go back to sleep." And we stay lying down, tossing and turning the night away. When we do wake up, of course, we feel terrible and groggy, but blame it on not sleeping well. Perhaps, however, we were merely sleeping too much!

As Soma and I thought about all these issues regarding sleep and the brain, I marveled at the fact that I had never heard any of it in medical school. Sleep was never discussed, except perhaps in some nostalgic way, since we all felt that we had had too little of it. Yet the subject is clearly extremely important. You cannot have an appreciation for the ebb and flow of our bodies' fluids throughout the day and night without appreciating the changes that we undergo each day as a result of gravity and the position in which we sleep. Despite the fact that these ideas are almost never discussed (except in space medicine), they are true to the principles of human anatomy and physiology.

What do they have to do with migraines?

Migraines are a vascular headache. They are characterized by pressure in the head. Arteries leading to the brain apparently contract, and then open widely, causing intense pressurizing of the brain. In addition, migraines are associated with excessive sleeping. People who experience migraines frequently report getting them after sleeping in late on the weekend. Could there be some connection between migraines and the head pressurizing that occurs during horizontal sleep time?

Intracranial Hypertension

Intracranial hypertension means high pressure in the brain. What is the effect of intracranial hypertension? The most common feature of intracranial hypertension is headache! It also includes nausea, vomiting, visual disturbances and weakness of the extremities. In fact, it sounds just like a migraine.

Increased pressure in, or on, the veins leading down from the brain and into the heart can lead to increased intracranial pressure. This increased vein pressure can be caused by such behaviors as coughing, straining, and crying, or it can happen from chronic heart failure. Obstruction of the jugular veins or of the superior vena cava, which are the large veins entering the heart from the head, can cause increased pressure in the brain. Increased carbon dioxide in the blood increases the brain's blood supply and blood pressure by opening up resistance arterioles in the brain, thereby increasing cerebral spinal fluid pressure and brain pressure. These facts are commonly known in medicine.

What is considered to be the most common cause of intracranial hypertension? It has been assumed to be a tumor, since the tumor may obstruct the normal pathway of the cerebral spinal fluid or the venous drainage of blood from the brain, resulting in fluid build-up and pressure. Another cause is a condition termed pseudotumor cerebri, meaning a false tumor. It refers to increased intracranial pressure in the absence of a tumor or other obvious obstruction of the cerebral spinal fluid pathway. The cause is usually not discovered, although it is thought to involve reduced venous drainage of the brain. Its symptoms? Headache, visual disturbances, vomiting, vertigo, ringing in the ears. These signs are considered to arise from the shifts of normal brain structures caused by the increased intracranial pressure.

These conditions, a brain tumor and pseudotumor cerebri, both resemble migraines in their manifestation. It would be hard to differentiate between these conditions, which is why people who experience migraines for the first time are checked by their neurologist for a brain tumor. Could there be another, more common cause of this pressure that has been ignored and that might lead to all these conditions? Nothing is ever mentioned about sleep and gravity!

Too Flat for Too Long

A theory began to emerge, and it was a testable theory. We imagined the following scenario.

From childhood, people develop sleeping patterns, including length of time asleep and position of sleep. If their habits are such that they result in excessive pressurizing of the head, there will be congestion of the brain, or brain edema, which may at first have no signs or symptoms apart from slight lethargy and occasional headache. Of course, since we get used to our sleeping habits and patterns, we become accustomed to how we feel as a result of those patterns. So we may never recognize what our patterns of sleep are doing to us, having no frame of reference with which to compare.

Let's assume that this edema, which is difficult to clear from the brain due to lack of lymphatics, never completely goes away during the vertical time of our waking day. This would lead to chronic edema, and the slow, progressive choking of the brain tissue. One early morning, perhaps after a particularly stressful day when the brain is tired, and after sleeping most of the night, the brain is stimulated. Perhaps it is by a particularly exciting dream, or by a sound in the street, or a smell in the air. The brain needs oxygen and sugar when stimulated. However, the oxygen in the brain is low due to the chronic edema, which prevents tissue reoxygenation. The sugar level in the brain is low, too, due to the overexertion of the tissue and the edema. And the carbon dioxide level is high. In response, the brain signals for its arterioles to open up.

The only way that the brain is going to get what it needs is from the blood. And the only way to get the blood is to increase the pressure. The pressure in the brain does rise, but this leads to further edema. It is not simply a matter of getting the blood into the brain. There must also be drainage of blood from the brain to allow circulation. Circulation of the fluid is what is needed, not simply pressurizing the brain further. Stagnant tissue will remain stagnant despite pressure. What is needed is circulation to flush out the old and bring in the new. However, the drainage is impaired, since gravity cannot pull down on the blood in the head while the head is in a horizontal position.

Migraines as a Brain Flush

At this point, the pressure inside the brain may lead to dysfunction, resulting in auras and other neurological manifestations of the so-called migraine "prodrome", which is a term referring to the early signs of the migraine. To manage the crisis, the brain may elicit what we call a *migraine response* as an emergency flush. The carotid arteries open widely as do the arterioles and the entire brain slowly forces itself to flush under the pressure of the heart pumping blood through it. This is painful, but essential to preserve the brain. Meanwhile the brain makes sure that it is left alone with no stimulation, lowering its need for oxygen and sugar. It does this by making sure its body stays in bed, lights out, in a quiet room, preferably asleep.

Eventually, flushed and out of its crisis, the arteries stop dilating and return to a normal diameter. The migraine has ended and the brain has been saved, but the cause of the chronic edema has not been eliminated. So long as the brain's edema and need for nutrients and oxygen can be managed, the migraine is not needed. But as soon as the brain gets over stimulated, undernourished, and over-congested, it may elicit another migraine response.

In brief, our theory is that migraines are the body's defense mechanism to flush a congested, starving brain. Why does it usually occur on one side of the head? Most people sleep on their side. Gravity still affects the horizontal brain, making the down side get more fluid than the up side of the brain. This asymmetry would cause one side to be more congested than the other. The brain may autoregulate its flushing mechanism to preferentially flush the more congested side. Alternatively, both sides may be equally flushed, but the chronically more congested side will feel it more, since it is already more congested and swollen.

Explaining Other Migraine Findings

This theory can explain several findings that have been a source of confusion for those trying to understand migraines.

- *Women have more migraines than men, and typically have them near the time of their menstrual period.*

It is before a woman's menstrual period that her levels of the hormone estrogen are the highest. This hormone increases the retention of fluid in the body, which causes the puffiness and discomfort of Pre-Menstrual Syndrome. It also can raise the blood pressure. During this time, then, women have a greater than usual fluid pressure in their bodies, including in their brains. This no doubt also explains the irritability associated with this time of the month. If an already congested brain is made even more congested by estrogen, the edema worsens, and the conditions become ripe for a migraine. Oral contraceptives and estrogen replacement also can increase migraine incidence and severity. The only time estrogen does not seem to be a problem is during late pregnancy. However, at this time there is an increased blood sugar level, which, as you will see below, can help a sugar starved brain and prevent some migraines.

- *It is generally thought that there is a genetic component to migraines, but no definitive pattern of inheritance has been found.*

It is always difficult to differentiate between a trait inherited through one's genes, and a trait learned through one's family-trained habits. If migraines run in a family it could simply be because of familial sleeping patterns. Parents accustomed to sleeping long hours will possibly expect their children to do the same. If a parent sleeps flat on his or her stomach, children may copy this behavior, or may simply become conditioned to sleeping in that position by having been placed down in the crib that way. Later in the book we will show how various sleeping positions can affect the brain and body.

There might be certain inherited problems with brain drainage pathways and blood vessel connections that reduce brain circulation, worsening the gravity effect. However, these would be rare, and they certainly have not been identified for migraines. This makes sleep behavior training a more likely explanation for why migraines can run in families.

- *Vomiting can quickly end a child's migraine.*

Vomiting temporarily creates a tremendous increase in blood pressure. The position of the head while vomiting is level with or lower than the heart, making the blood pressure temporarily high in the brain. This effectively forces blood through the brain. Vomiting, then, may be a natural mechanism for a quick brain flush.

- *Stress provokes migraines after the stressful event has ended.*

Stress increases the body's need for oxygen and nutrients. After the stressful event, the body may be depleted of these vital substances. If the brain is already chronically congested with edema from flat sleep posture, it will be difficult to oxygenate the brain tissue and deliver the needed sugar for proper brain functioning. A stressful event, then, may deplete the body of the substances that the brain already needs, eliciting a migraine response.

- *Exercise prevents migraines.*

Exercise increases overall body and brain circulation and increases respiration. This can help flush and oxygenate a congested brain, making a migraine response unnecessary.

- *Muscle stiffness after exercise can cause a migraine.*

Muscle stiffness is a sign of continuously contracting muscle fibers. Muscle fiber contraction requires sugar and oxygen. When you are exercising, increased circulation and breathing help deliver oxygen and sugar to the muscles. After exercising, however, the continued contraction of stiff muscles begins to rob the otherwise resting body of oxygen and sugar. This competes with the brain for these substances. If the brain is already needy, it could produce a migraine to get what it needs.

- *Events or substances that trigger migraines do not always trigger attacks in the same person.*

All that a trigger for a migraine does is stimulate the brain, which turns on various brain centers. This increases the brain's requirement for oxygen and sugar. Whether or not the stimulus will trigger a migraine at any given time depends not on the trigger, but on the state of the brain at that time. A congested brain may respond to the trigger with a migraine. If it is not too congested at the time, there may be no problem at all.

- *Fasting or insufficient food intake and insulin-induced low blood sugar can precipitate a migraine.*

One of the early signs that a migraine attack is coming is a craving for sweets. The brain's primary energy source is glucose, which is the sugar in our blood. If the sugar level in the brain is too low, it needs to get it from somewhere. It has virtually no stores of sugar, and the only place to get it is from the blood. Fasting and excessive insulin both cause low blood sugar, or hypoglycemia, further depriving the starved brain. Depending on how desperate the situation is for the brain, it may elicit a migraine response to get whatever sugar is available.

- *Muscle pain in the neck can trigger migraines.*

One of the results of stress is a tight neck. Poor posture, too much computer work, or sleeping the wrong way can create stiff neck muscles, as can accidents and injuries. Blood must flow through the neck to circulate to and from the brain. A tight neck restricts this circulation of blood, as the contracted, inflamed muscles impinge on nearby veins, arteries, and even nerves leading to and from the head. It is as though the tight muscles constrict the circulation from the inside. Of course, this lowers brain oxygen and sugar, in addition to hampering the nervous pathways. To cope with the reduced circulation, a migraine response may be needed.

Note that this may also explain part of the mechanism for tension headaches. The effect of tension on the brain may be an indirect result of neck tightness and its effect on brain circulation. Tension and tight necks are commonly associated.

- *Low oxygen at high altitudes and in decompression chambers produces migraines.*

The brain needs oxygen, just as it needs sugar. Some migraines can be stopped by supplying oxygen, indicating that a need for oxygen is part of the problem. Migraines are the brain's way of making sure that it gets what it needs.

- *Astronauts living in zero gravity get migraines.*

Zero gravity means that there is no gravity operating on the body, which is what happens in space. This is a similar situation to when the head and heart are on the same horizontal plane, as when lying flat. In both cases, gravity does not assist the drainage of blood from the brain, or resist the pumping of blood to the brain, leading to brain edema. Numerous studies have looked into this effect of zero gravity on the bodies of astronauts, and have studied this effect in laboratories on Earth by having subjects lie down flat. In other words, lying down flat has been used to simulate zero gravity. It has been discovered that the lack of gravity causes a shift of fluid from the body into the head, which causes brain edema. The result is a migraine, as well as other problems associated with brain congestion.[4]

We were amazed at how many features of migraines are explained by our theory. Fortunately, the theory is easily testable. That is important. It is one thing to come up with a theory. It is another thing to test it. The theory already passed the preliminary test of making sense out of a variety of phenomena associated with migraines. Now we had to test it directly.

We were elated. We told Camela what to do. It was something we would study on migraineurs as the ultimate test of the theory. If we were correct, they might never have to suffer from migraines again.

4

The Migraine Relief Project

It is at this point in a research project that you have to be careful that you are not simply trying to prove a point. Actually, you are supposed to challenge your hypothesis by exposing it to rigorous tests. You should be trying to prove yourself wrong.

Considering the Variables

Realize that research into migraines never can consider all possible variables. No research could, since the nature of research is to discover those very variables. Migraine research, in addition, has always ignored this variable of gravity on brain circulation. Variables such as estrogen fluctuations, blood pressure changes throughout the day, sleeping behavior, and diet are usually ignored in migraine studies, unless they are the focus of the study itself. However, while it is the nature of research to ignore some variables, you cannot ignore those that are central to the process you are studying and expect to get meaningful results. Ignoring gravity and sleep behavior has been a fatal flaw in migraine research to date.

In fact, the migraine literature is extremely contradictory and confused. Argument still rages over whether or not classic migraine, with aura, is the same phenomenon as common migraine, which does not have an aura. There is disagreement over the nature of the pain in the brain, since most brain tissue, except for the thalamus, hypothalamus, and membranes covering the brain, feel no pain. Experts are in conflict over the exact mechanism of the migraine attack. Is it caused by the blood vessels, or by some substances in the blood, or by the nervous tissue of the brain itself? Over 100 years of research has not cleared up the issue. What could be the problem?

Dissection versus Connection

One problem is that modern medical research is typically an analytic process that divides and dissects the whole of our bodies into minute parts, each of which gets studied by a specialist. As these specialists focus more and more on their limited, dissected worlds, they can easily lose sight of the whole picture.

The brain, for example, cannot be dissected into vessels, fluid, and nervous tissue without losing sight that it is one, integrated organ. You cannot understand a part out of the context of its whole. Indeed, you cannot understand the brain without considering the rest of the body, to which that brain belongs. What happens in the lungs, or the penis, or the heart will affect the brain. It's all connected.

Taking this line of reasoning further, we see that you cannot really understand the body without understanding the culture, which conditions the attitudes and behaviors of that body. We are more than a body. We are people. More than that, we are a certain culture of people. Our culture defines all we think, do, and say. It can alter our anatomy and physiology. You cannot understand human health and disease without examining this greater cultural whole of which we all are a small part.

Modern science is focused on making distinctions. This makes it difficult for scientists to make connections. When you have a jigsaw puzzle in front of you, it is better to connect the pieces than it is to cut up each piece into even smaller fragments. Yet, this has been the dominant research strategy regarding migraines.

The Heisenberg Uncertainty Principle

In addition to the confusion that this "divide and conquer" mentality creates, there is another problem inherent in brain research, which is insurmountable. It relates to the Heisenberg Uncertainty Principle. This principle, defined by the German physicist Heisenberg in the 1930's, addresses the impossibility of simultaneously determining the exact position and momentum of a sub-atomic particle. In other words, when something as small as an electron, for example, is studied to find its position and direction of movement, you cannot help but interfere with its movement and position by that study. This translates into the generalization that you cannot study a system without changing it at the same time. When you check a battery to determine its charge, for another example, the process of checking the charge discharges some of the battery. All studies interfere with the subject that they are studying, unless you are engaging in some abstract mathematical or statistical research. When it comes to studying electrons and other sub-atomic particles, their minute size makes them extremely vulnerable to changes brought on by the experiment itself.

This same principle applies to medical tests. For example, when people get their blood pressure checked, the stress of the event can elevate the blood pressure. The mere operation of having a cuff pumped up tightly around your arm while sitting in a hospital hallway may elicit a higher blood pressure than you would normally have. Just waiting in an emergency room for a health care provider to look at you can raise your blood pressure. In short, you cannot determine blood pressure without altering it at the same time.

When it comes to the brain, this principle is also operative. The brain is not only a biological organ. It is the seat of our awareness. You cannot study the circulation of the brain of a person having a migraine without affecting that circulation by the

37

study itself. For example, researchers interested in studying brain circulation in people with migraines have frequently done so by injecting a special dye, which can be followed by a certain machine, into the neck arteries and watching the distribution of the dye as it courses throughout the brain. These dyes are known to have the potential for creating irritations within the blood vessels, and sometimes can result in a life-threatening allergic response. In addition, stabbing the carotid artery of the neck with a needle to inject the dye can possibly create spasms within the artery and the neck.

Imagine being the subject in this research. If someone was studying your brain circulation and approached your neck with a needle to inject dye into your carotid artery, would it alter your brain's circulation? Of course it would. Could you understand the usual brain circulation of a person under these stressful research conditions? The Uncertainty Principle says, "Certainly not!"

When you are researching the brain you alter it, since it is aware that you are doing research on it. This is a reflection of the Uncertainty Principle. Even in a broader sense this principle applies. You cannot dissect a whole into parts without altering what you have dissected. What you end up studying may simply be a product of your particular way of slicing up the whole. It may have nothing to do with the whole at all.

Studying Chemicals

Another problem with migraine research is that it reduces human nature to chemical reactions. For example, it is known that certain foods, such as chocolate, can trigger a migraine for some people. If you thought of people as real, whole beings, a product of both their culture and experience, you would think of food as more than a chemical substance. Food has cultural and personal significance. It reminds us of past experiences and associations with that food. It stimulates our mouths and nostrils, and begins a cascade of bodily digestive functions. Obtaining and preparing the food for consumption and anticipating how it will feel to eat is all part of the food experience. This is no less the case with chocolate than it is for other foods. In fact, chocolate often elicits an emotional response. People may eat it when depressed to make them feel better. It can even be addictive. In short, chocolate is a powerful stimulant of our brains, indeed, of our entire being.

To study chocolate as a trigger of migraines, researchers ignored this human element and went straight for the chemistry.[5] They assumed that if chocolate was a trigger, then there must be some chemical substance(s) in the chocolate that could be identified as such. To test this, they pumped chocolate directly into the stomachs of migraine sufferers who reported a chocolate trigger, ignoring the fact that people who get migraines from chocolate usually eat it instead of pumping it down. The researchers used a nasogastric tube that was inserted in the subject's nose and passed down into the stomach. Interestingly, the researchers found the pumped in chocolate did not trigger a migraine. This left many people confused, since it defied a chemical explanation as to why chocolate may be a migraine trigger. Too bad they were only focusing on chemistry, and not on people.

Studying Animals

Sometimes, this neglect of the human factor gets migraine research into even more ridiculous situations, as when studies are performed on rats, mice, or other non-humans. It should be obvious that you cannot interpret the signs of a migraine on a rodent, for example. A rat cannot tell you about the pain in its head, or describe auras. We cannot even be certain that they get migraines. This creates a problem for animal researchers who need to somehow model a migraine on a rodent or other creature. How can you give a mouse a migraine? And what does this possibly tell you about the cause of human migraines?

Even if you cause brain edema in the poor animal, its brain is not a human brain. It has a different anatomy and, therefore, a different physiology. Particularly significant with regards to the gravity issue, animals that have their heads almost always horizontal with respect to their bodies do not have to deal with the human issue of the effect of gravity while in the vertical versus the horizontal positions. If you use primates to better imitate the human posture, it still ignores the cultural conditioning of sleeping behaviors. In short, human diseases, particularly those caused by lifestyle or culture, must be studied in humans.

Studying Cells

Many researchers recognize the limits of animal research in predicting human response. Instead of using animals, some researchers use tissue culture. Cells from some person are removed from the body and placed in a Petri dish in liquid medium to allow the cells to grow. Studies are then performed on these cells, perhaps giving them new drugs, to see what happens. This is called in vitro, or in glass, research. The results of these tissue culture studies are known to not necessarily apply to the body as a whole. It may be, for example, that the substance tested on the tissue culture would be altered in the whole body, say, by the liver, making its affect on a whole, living organism different from that on a dish of cells. Scientists know this limitation of in vitro research. Yet, many spend their careers performing this research and trying to apply it to migraines, which may do nothing more than add confusing literature to the annals of medicine.

Creating Research Artifacts

All that this type of research generates is artifacts of its own experimental model and design. That is why so much migraine research, and brain research in general, is contradictory and inconclusive. What is being studied is not the brain and how it works, but the effects of the different research methods used to study the brain. Each researcher has his or her own method and focus, some preferring cells, others preferring guinea pigs, and others interested only in brain chemicals. The result has been over a century of conflicting theories and counter-theories about migraines.

Applied Medical Anthropology

We must deal with uncertainty, then, when studying rats instead of humans; or when studying cells apart from the organism from which they were derived; or when studying blood vessels and fluids and chemicals apart from the organs through which they circulate; or when studying brains apart from their bodies, or bodies apart from their culture. The only way out of this uncertainty is to reverse the process. We must not divide the whole into parts. We must reconnect the parts into a whole.

This is the essence of our applied medical anthropology approach. We try to look at the big picture, hoping to get big answers. In this big picture, we see people as a product of their culture, instead of seeing people as a product of their cells and biomolecules. We study how changes in attitude and behavior can alter our health. We use no drugs, dyes, surgery, or any invasive procedure. We simply ask people to try a simple, cost-free and risk-free lifestyle change, and then see what happens.

The Migraine Relief Project

As we began our Migraine Relief Project we expected that our research design might create some false negative results, or times when the migraines may have gone away but didn't, because of confounding variables. However, we knew that if the theory were correct, then the results would show it.

We conducted tests in Victoria, British Columbia, Canada, and in Hilo, Hawaii. To find participants, we advertised for migraine sufferers who wished to participate in a risk-free and cost-free study of the effects of lifestyle on migraines. The response to the ads was very positive. We screened applicants to find those with at least one migraine per month. Most of the participants had had migraines several times a week. All had had a diagnosis of migraines from a physician, and had been under medications at one time or another, which never had rid them of the migraines. The ages varied from the teens to the sixties. Most participants were female, but about 5% were male.

We interviewed the participants on the phone to determine their eligibility and interest in participating. Our method of doing applied medical anthropology research is to identify a lifestyle that we wish to study, explain our theory to participants, and describe how they are to alter their behavior for the study. The participants are supposed to record their progress, which we discuss with them over the phone at weekly intervals. The participants are also instructed not to alter any other behaviors over the study period, including taking any new drugs, and are to report any such irregularities at the time of the phone check-up.

The Lifestyle Change

The lifestyle change that we were researching was the effect of head elevation while sleeping. Sleeping flat pressurizes the head. Sleeping with the head slightly inclined allows better head drainage and circulation. Over time this may reduce head edema and eliminate the brain's need for a migraine response.

We offered the participants two alternatives for raising their beds. They could either use a foam wedge specially designed for the purpose of raising the head in bed. Or they could put some pillows or a sleeping bag between the box spring and mattress at the head of the bed. They were instructed to keep the foot of the bed level with the ground to prevent fluid accumulation in the feet. After all, horizontal time is needed by the feet and legs to lose their fluid while the head is getting re-pressurized. We indicated that everyone will feel comfortable at a different head elevation, and suggested that the top of the mattress should be elevated above the box spring by about 8 to 12 inches to achieve a 20-30 degree elevation. This would allow everyone to find his or her own comfortable height. In addition, they were allowed to use their regular pillow, raising their head height a bit more.

None of the study participants had been sleeping with their head elevated at the time of the study. The 3-month study began with 104 subjects. The test group, which was instructed to elevate their heads, consisted of 68 people. The control group, which slept normally, consisted of 36 people. At the time of the first week phone check-up we discovered that 8 people could not fulfill their promise to raise their beds, and they dropped out of the study. We also discovered at that time that 8 more participants in the test group were too uncomfortable sleeping elevated, so they were placed in the control group. Over the rest of the 3 months, the test group remained at 52 and the control group at 44 subjects.

The Results

What we found was significant and clear. Some people in the test group immediately reported having the best night of sleep they had had in years. Others felt results by three weeks into the study. In total, by the end of the study, 16 people stopped having migraines. An additional 20 people experienced fewer and less severe migraines, allowing them to avoid taking any medications to deal with the pain. This means that 36 people were helped by raising their beds. The control group consisted of 44 people, and one person in that group experienced a spontaneous recovery. So we can still assume that virtually all of the test subjects who recovered did so because of the head elevation. However, it did not work for everyone, with 16 people in the test group reporting no improvement.

This means that 36 out of 52 people in the test group responded to the head elevation, which is about 70% of the total. And about 30% fully lost their migraines.

Confounding Variables

Why did some participants continue to have headaches? People who suffer from migraines, as we have said, also may suffer from tension headaches, which may be difficult to differentiate from a migraine. So some of our participants may have lost their migraines due to raising their beds, but may nevertheless have experienced a tension headache, which may have a different mechanism of action that is less dependent on head elevation. This would work against the theory seeming correct, since it would create reports of headaches that could be interpreted as migraines, although they were not. For the study we assumed that all the headaches participants experienced during the study period were migraines.

Another problem is ensuring that the participant stayed on the inclined portion of their bed without sliding down the incline. Camela, for example, was sleeping on a foam wedge that was specially designed for head elevation. Yet, each morning we would see her in bed curled at the bottom of the wedge into a fetal position, her head flat against the horizontal mattress. Sleeping behaviors are difficult to change. It is hard for people to monitor their behavior while sleeping. This means that some of the participants who elevated their beds did not necessarily stay on the elevated part, and, therefore, did not benefit from the elevation.

We also did not control for side sleeping versus back sleeping. Side sleeping is known to reduce brain circulation and increase brain pressure and edema. (See references) Those who did not get rid of migraines by head elevation may have spent more time side sleeping.

Several people in the study developed backaches and neck aches as a result of changing their head elevation. We instructed them to use a pillow under the back of their knees to bend the legs and reduce back strain. This helped in some cases. However, some people could not feel comfortable sleeping elevated. These issues led us to withdraw some people from the test group and place them in the control group, as we mentioned.

It is also possible, as a confounding variable in this study, that head elevation may not fully compensate for such factors as neck tightness and constrictive clothing and jewelry. Tight neck muscles can impair blood flow to and from the head, as we discuss in more detail later. The improvement afforded by head elevation during sleep can be negated, at least in part, by a tight neck. Clothing, such as neckties around tightly collared shirts, can act like a tourniquet, choking the circulation to and from the head during the day. Tight necklaces, heavy gold chains around the neck, and fashionable choker collars can also interfere with head circulation. All these factors can minimize the positive effect of head elevation on migraines since they make the congestion worse by interfering with gravity drainage of the head during the day.

The use of pillows can create another problem. A pillow can press into the side of the neck, hampering the blood supply to and drainage from the brain. In addition, sleeping position, such as sleeping with the head to the side, can cause the impingement of arteries and veins in the neck, resulting in poor brain circulation.

Then there is the possibility that the body may retain fluid due to changes in hormones during the study period. We have already discussed how estrogen can increase bodily fluid and thereby create greater edema in the head, making migraines more likely. Additionally, any cause of increased blood pressure, or hypertension, can congest the head and further predispose a person to a migraine. This cause could be high stress, high estrogen, high salt in the diet, as well as disease conditions affecting the heart, blood vessels, or kidneys. Any of these factors may have masked benefits from the head elevation effect that we were trying to study.

Addictions and Withdrawals

Many of the participants were also regular migraine drug users, and headaches can result from addiction to and withdrawal from these drugs. This relationship between headaches and pharmaceutical drugs is frequently misunderstood. For example, many people believe that caffeine is useful in ridding oneself of a headache. Caffeine is known to be a vasoconstrictor, closing down the blood vessels going to the brain. This lowers the pressure of the fluid entering the brain, reducing the pain of the headache. It is for this reason that caffeine is included in many migraine medications. However, what is not realized is that caffeine withdrawal creates headaches. Caffeine, of course, is in coffee, certain teas, and cola beverages. It is added to some non-cola beverages to give an extra kick to the drink. And it is highly addictive, which helps the sales of these products. The brain gets used to the constrictive effect of the caffeine, and a rebound effect happens when caffeine is withdrawn, causing vasodilation. This increases fluid pressure in the brain, and results in a headache. So caffeine can create headaches by conditioning the brain to get used to its vasoconstrictive effects, causing headaches on its withdrawal. More caffeine at those times may stop the rebound vasodilation effect, but it is hard to credit the caffeine for stopping the headache when addiction to caffeine may have been the cause of the problem in the first place. It may be difficult, then, to rule out headaches due to chemical substance use, abuse, and withdrawal during the study period, which can again mask the positive effect of head elevation.

Vasoconstrictive drugs have been the mainstay of migraine treatment. As with caffeine, they can have a rebound effect upon withdrawal, creating another headache. In fact, headaches can be a side effect of migraine medications. This creates an interesting dilemma. If someone takes a drug for a headache, but the drug can itself cause a headache, then the next headache that that person experiences could be from the drug, and not from the cause of the original headache. If that person then takes the same drug for that second headache, they will enter into a cycle of headaches that follows their pill cycle. At that point the person may begin to think that he or she has a headache problem, when in actuality it's a drug problem.

All of these confounding variables were at play to one extent or another in our study. However, their combined effect makes head elevation seem less beneficial that it may be. This means that our results may have been even more positive had everyone stayed elevated, had loose neck muscles, had not experienced drug withdrawal or tension headaches, etc. Yet, despite these interferences with the elevation effect, 70% reported success with this lifestyle change.

Experimental Controls

Does this lack of standardization between participants invalidate the study? Must we control for all the above variables to make any sense out of the results? Let's consider the results. If a study participant stopped having headaches it can mean one of three possibilities: the condition may have disappeared all by itself; or the participant's own expectations and faith in the process resulted in recovery due to the placebo effect; or the head elevation really did work. Let's examine these three possibilities in turn.

Spontaneous recovery, in which the migraines stop without apparent intervention, was measured in our study by using a control group. You always need a control group, which is a group of subjects that does nothing new. If a certain percentage of this group recovers without any intervention, then you can assume that a similar percentage of the test group would have done the same. You then have to subtract the percentage of incidences of spontaneous recovery within the control group from the percentage recovering within the test group. It could be that some unknown variables were responsible for the spontaneous recovery. But that constitutes another research question. All you have to do is give the test group a new behavior and ask them to change nothing else. Then have a control group that simply changes nothing. At the end you see if the change in the test group was helpful or not, compared to the control group.

As we stated, only one person out of the 44 in the control group experienced a spontaneous recovery. This means that we can assume that spontaneous recovery is not a significant variable in this study.

Next to consider is the placebo effect. This refers to the fact that people heal better when they believe in the treatment given. The treatment is only part of the cure. The other part is caused by the person's faith in the treatment that stimulates the internal healing processes that leads to the cure. This placebo effect plays a part in all disease treatment. The healing power of the mind affects the outcome of the treatment.

In drug research you control for the placebo effect by giving the control group a sugar pill instead of the drug. The sugar pill is supposed to have no physiological effects. The subjects taking the sugar pill, however, think that they are taking the drug, leading to a placebo response. In this way you can tell the degree to which psychological expectations alter the biological effects of a drug.

To what degree did the placebo effect alter our results? We couldn't have given a sugar pill, but we could have asked some participants to alter an insignificant sleeping behavior that has nothing to do with gravity and body position, to see how many recovered simply due to an expectation that they would recover. However, we felt that this was unnecessary for a preliminary study, especially since all the participants were veteran migraineurs who had no recovery from years of drug therapy. We assumed that if years of therapy by their doctors could not elicit a placebo mediated recovery in these people, then our study would not, either. However, larger follow-up studies should consider this factor in the research design.

If we can rule out spontaneous recovery and placebo effects, then chances are that the 70% response rate in the study was a result of the lifestyle change tested. We felt that the results would be significant and obvious if the theory were correct, since we were examining a possible mechanism for migraines. Confounding variables may hide a small factor. A large causative factor will make itself known.

Changing Sleeping Behavior

We were most able to study Camela, since she was living in our house. I could see her resistance to sleeping elevated, since it was a new experience for her. Many people in the study, in fact, did not want to change their sleeping behavior. It is one of those things we have done since the womb. People find an escape in their sleep. This was especially true for Camela. She would sleep 10-12 hours nightly, and would have slept more if we had let her. I believe that she was depressed emotionally, which is not unusual for someone who suffers from excruciating, recurrent headaches. Sleep seemed to be her time to rest from her pain and fears. Ironically, her sleep was causing her problems in the first place.

Her improvement was slight in the beginning. We then observed her sleeping and noticed that she was not staying on the incline plane. She resisted our coaching and insistence that she keep her head elevated, but she did finally learn to elevate her head. Soon her migraines subsided in intensity. Then they disappeared.

When you get these results from a preliminary study, you know that you are onto something big. Realize that we may have had even more amazing results if we had controlled for many of the variables we discussed above. This makes head elevation a very significant factor in migraines, and supports our theory that gravity and sleep behavior are the keys.

Follow-up Studies

Naturally, one study is not definitive. We hope that this study could be repeated in a sleep research facility, where people can be monitored as they sleep to determine length of time down, degree of head elevation, and whether or not they stay elevated without sliding to the side of the bed or down to the bottom of the incline plane. Additionally, it is important to note how the subject is sleeping. Are they sleeping on the side, with a nostril closed, or on the back, with both nostrils open? This might affect brain function and the creation of migraines.

Nevertheless, we were elated with the findings. Migraines had never been connected with head pressure upon lying down to sleep, until now. Could this be the light at the end of the tunnel for migraine sufferers? Is it possible that there is more to this gravity connection? Could it help explain some other mysteries of brain dysfunction?

5

The Missing Link

This chapter is a bit technical, since it deals with several health conditions, their features, and their connections to one another. The issues are really simple to understand. However, the language of medicine is designed to make the simple complex. How else can medical researchers and doctors call themselves "experts", particularly when they admit to having no answers as to the cause, or cure, of these conditions? Confusing language merely provides the needed mystique. We have tried to cut through the façade, and encourage the lay reader to press on.

Most of what we are about to share with you is standard medical information that you can find in any general medical textbook, and we provide generous reference support in the appendix. What we have added to the picture is the factor of gravity and sleep position in understanding the cause of these conditions and their relationship to one another. It will make it seem as though the cause of migraines, stroke, Alzheimer's, glaucoma, and other brain conditions, as well as impotence, should have been known all along. Medical researchers have not made these connections since they consider these conditions to be separate entities. They are busy defining the differences between these diseases, instead of finding their common cause.

Summary

We have shown that elevation of the head during sleeping can stop migraines from occurring. The proposed mechanism, as we have explained, is that the gravity assisted drainage of the brain, as well as the gravity resisted pressurizing of the head, are the result of standing, when the heart is below the head. Once a person lies down to sleep, this effect of gravity is lost, leading to increased arterial pressure into the brain and reduced venous drainage from the brain. In other words, the brain drains when we stand or sit erect, and pressurizes with fluid when we lie down to sleep. Given the length of time a person remains in the horizontal position, and how flat they are when lying down, the relationship between head drainage and head pressurizing can become uneven, so that there is net head pressurization. This may become a chronic, or long-standing condition, with the time spent each day in the vertical, upright position unable to compensate for the increased brain pressure generated when lying down.

This condition of increased brain fluid is called edema, and its features are decreased oxygen and sugar in the brain, higher carbon dioxide, and greater mechanical pressure exerted on internal brain structures. Stimulation of the brain, or a "trigger", causes an increased demand for oxygen and sugar, which an edematous brain is already lacking. In response, the brain's autoregulatory mechanism causes the arteries in the neck and brain to dilate, allowing greater flow of blood to the brain in the hope of flushing out the depleted tissue. This is the migraine response, and it subsides once the brain has flushed itself.

What happens if the migraine response does not happen, or if the brain is repeatedly congested? If this model of migraines were correct, then there would be other diseases caused by brain edema, and somehow related to migraines. Indeed, when you search the medical literature it is clear that migraines are connected to many other brain diseases, all of which might respond well, and may be preventable, by decreasing head pressure through elevating the head of the bed while sleeping.

Stroke

Let us begin with one of the major killers of our time — stroke. A stroke is a type of cerebrovascular disease, which is a disorder of the arteries or veins of the brain or of their contents. The term "stroke" refers to the functional brain injury resulting from the disease process. The cause of the stroke can be low oxygen and nutrients in the brain due to a problem associated with the circulatory system within the head, creating an ischemic stroke. Or it can be due to abnormal leakage of blood into or around brain structures, creating a hemorrhagic stroke. Let us now consider the first cause just mentioned.

Ischemic Stroke

Ischemia simply means reduced blood flow. When blood cannot get to the brain, tissues starve of oxygen and a lack of sugar, and can begin to die. What can inhibit blood from getting to those parts of the brain? It could be due to a thrombus, or clot, getting lodged in the smaller arteries within the brain. The part of the brain where that artery was supposed to carry blood suffers, as the clot clogs the vessel and shuts off the blood supply. Once tissue oxygen goes below 40 mm of Hg the cells can no longer survive. A simple blood clot is one of the major causes of clogs in the arteries. Arterial clots are the result of some damage within the lining of the blood vessels or the heart. The clot breaks apart and a piece is sent with the blood into the brain, only to become stuck in the vessel as the diameter gets smaller, blocking the rest of that vessel's pathway.

In addition to clots clogging the arteries, there can also be trouble from plaques lining the carotid arteries to the brain, a condition called atherosclerosis. These plaques can break off and lodge further down the vascular pathway, which, for the carotids, is up in the head. Even bacterial plaques from a diseased heart valve can create an embolism, or plug, to cause an infarction, which is an area of tissue destruction caused by a plugged blood vessel.

A clot in the veins, however, is different. It can form by platelets in the blood simply clumping together. Platelets are tiny cellular fragments that circulate in the blood. They contain enzymes for the clotting of blood, and assisting in blood clotting is their key function. However, when blood pools and is low in oxygen, platelets spontaneously clump together, creating what is called a venous thrombosis, or a clot in the veins. This happens in the legs in individuals with poor venous drainage from those limbs. This is why phlebitis, which is an inflammation of the veins, can lead to dangerous blood clots. Valves within the leg veins usually direct blood upwards, against gravity, to return it to the heart. When these valves become damaged, perhaps by phlebitis, the veins lose their gravity defying ability, causing blood pooling and clot formation. This increases tissue fluid pressure, creating edema. Of course, this edema may ultimately progress to tissue degeneration if it becomes chronic.

Blood in the brain may pool in the venous sinuses, particularly due to a lack of gravity drainage when the body is horizontal in bed. This pooling, combined with the low oxygen content of the blood in the brain due to chronic edema, can cause the blood to clot, creating what is called a cerebral venous sinus thrombosis. This will create a further obstruction to the drainage of the brain, leading to a stroke. Remember that it is not just an issue of getting blood into the brain that counts. It is brain circulation that is needed. Circulation requires drainage of blood out from the head, not just increased delivery of blood into the head.

In addition, chronic brain edema from lying flat increases brain tissue pressure, which may possibly lead to impingement of the brain capillaries. It is hard for blood to flow through swollen tissue, making it more likely that a clot or plaque will lodge within a vessel, creating a stroke.

Brain tumor compression on surrounding tissue can obstruct blood vessels, as can plaques within the blood vessels, and these are the causes of ischemia that doctors typically look for in their diagnosis. The effect of gravity is completely ignored in all discussions of the causes of ischemia, yet it clearly is a major factor in brain blood flow. Lying flat minimizes brain circulation, as we have described, which has the same effect as an obstruction to blood flow. An ischemic stroke, then, may result from the same gravity issue that creates migraines.

Ischemia and Edema

In ischemia, blood is not adequately perfusing the brain, causing lower oxygen and sugar and higher carbon dioxide levels in the brain tissue. Edema creates the same problem. One of the damaging features of a stroke is its creation of further edema. The edema denies the surrounding tissue of oxygen extending the damage of the stroke to adjacent brain areas.

One outcome of ischemia and edema is deterioration of blood vessels. The cells lining the inside of blood vessels need oxygen and nutrients, too, but are deprived of these under ischemic and edematous conditions. The possible result of this is breakdown of the blood vessel integrity, leading to cerebrovascular disease. These diseased blood vessels can clot and clog, causing a stroke.

Stroke and Migraines

Stroke victims can experience many of the same symptoms as migraine sufferers. Both can get unilateral headaches, visual disturbances, unilateral face and body numbness and tingling, and other shared neurological dysfunctions. They are clearly both related to the same phenomenon, namely, poor brain circulation and brain edema and the resulting reduction in brain oxygen and sugar levels.

Generalized edema is related to high intracranial pressure, as we have discussed. One type of ischemic stroke is called hypertensive encephalopathy, which means a disease of the brain due to high blood pressure. This is an extreme situation of brain hypertension, but the mode of its operation also relates to that of migraines. High pressure in the arteries from the heart causes the brain's arterioles to constrict, in an attempt to minimize the excess pressure. In hypertensive encephalopathy the blood pressure that needs to be managed is too great for the brain's autoregulatory mechanism to cope. Some arterioles shut down to resist pressure, while others open up in response to high carbon dioxide levels in the tissue, in an attempt to get more oxygen. So a combination of extreme vasoconstriction and vasodilation occurs in different parts of the brain, leading to some areas of too much blood pressure in the brain, causing bleeding, and other areas of too little blood, causing ischemia. What are the symptoms? They are similar to a migraine — headache, nausea, vomiting, and, sometimes, cortical blindness. It can even cause seizures, which we will return to in a moment. By the way, cerebral venous sinus thrombosis, which we explained is the clotting of blood in the venous sinuses in the brain, has similar symptoms as hypertensive encephalopathy. This should be no surprise, since clots in the veins that descend from the brain to the heart prevent fluid drainage, leading to a back up of cerebral spinal fluid and blood in the brain and creating brain edema and ischemia. If blood cannot get out of the brain, then the new, fresh blood cannot get in, either. Again, migraines are clearly related to this same phenomenon of brain congestion and pressure, but to a lesser degree than in ischemic stroke.

Cortical Blindness

We mentioned something called cortical blindness as a symptom of hypertensive encephalopathy. This interesting condition refers to blindness caused by the brain's interpretation of visual information, not to blindness caused by something wrong with the eyes. The part of the brain responsible for receiving visual input from the eyes is the occipital part of the cerebral cortex, located on the rear part of the brain. Prizefighters may become blind from punches to the face, causing the back of the brain, the occipital area, to bang into the skull, damaging these visual centers of the cerebrum and creating cortical blindness. Apart from this type of head trauma, temporary cortical blindness is caused by three major conditions: insufficient blood delivered to that part of the brain; hypertensive encephalopathy; and – migraines!

Stroke and Sleep

We have been discussing the relationship between migraines and ischemic stroke. All the conditions we have just discussed are subcategories of ischemic stroke. They all seem related to migraines. However, we have another important piece of evidence that relates migraines to ischemic stroke. When does ischemic stroke most often occur? It most commonly occurs during sleep!! No explanation is made of this fact in the medical literature. But we think we now know why. That's when people lie down and develop pressurized, congested brains.

Hemorrhagic Stroke

The other type of stroke, called hemorrhagic stroke, is caused by broken blood vessels in the brain and the damage resulting from bleeding into the brain tissues. The major cause of this type of stroke is progressive damage and final rupture of a brain blood vessel due to hypertension, atherosclerosis, or a degenerative disease of the arteries. Again we see hypertension as a culprit. Whenever we see too much blood pressure as a cause, it follows that the effect of gravity on head pressure is a factor. A lifelong habit of lying too flat for too long unrelentingly pressurizes brain arteries, which are notorious for being relatively devoid of elastic tissue in their walls. This makes it easy for an aneurysm to form, which is a ballooning out of the wall of the artery. When an aneurysm bursts, it leads to a hemorrhagic stroke. In addition, the brain edema from lying flat weakens the blood vessels, as we discussed, possibly leading to cerebrovascular disease. Besides the clots that this may cause, degeneration of the blood vessels makes them more likely to leak or rupture under pressure, resulting in a hemorrhagic stroke.

Preventing Strokes

Migraines, ischemic stroke, hemorrhagic stroke, and cerebral aneurysms all relate to circulatory problems within the brain. All can be caused by the gravity effect we have been discussing. It is known that treatment of hypertension after a first stroke can help prevent a second stroke. It is known that all brain dysfunctions arising from hypertension should have the hypertension reduced. However, the most obvious way to reduce brain hypertension is to elevate the head when sleeping. No drugs or surgery are required. Just raise the head and the pressure in the head goes down.

We should make clear that the above discussion relates the *cause* of migraines to the *cause* of strokes. This connection is new to medicine, since the cause of migraines is said to be unknown, and the gravity/sleep effect has been overlooked as a cause of brain edema. It is known, however, that a migraine attack can itself lead to a stroke. (See references) Increased intracranial pressure during the migraine response can be the last straw for a chronically edematous and pressurized brain. Head elevation, then, may prevent strokes directly, by lowering intracranial pressure and reducing brain edema, and indirectly, by eliminating the need for a migraine response.

Seizures

Let's return to other possible connections between brain problems and migraines. We mentioned seizures. The term "seizure" simply refers to an attack, usually of sudden onset. It refers to the observation that people who have seizures seem to suddenly be attacked by some strange force that results in uncontrollable and abnormal motor, sensory, or psychological behavior, and is associated with an abnormally hyperactive part of the brain. If the seizures are recurrent and chronic, it is called epilepsy. Many seizures, however, occur once in a while and are therefore not considered epilepsy.

The Fatigued Brain

What can cause these seizures? Certain areas of the brain seem to lose control and begin a cascade of electrical discharges that can spread to other areas of the brain. Brain cells operate and communicate with one another through chemical and electrical signals. When a section of brain tissue becomes depleted of oxygen and sugar it cannot maintain its integrity and self-control. You can see this phenomenon in human behavior. When someone starts to get tired, especially a child, the energy necessary for self-control is lost first, and the person becomes agitated and hyperactive. Once this energy is spent, they finally settle down and rest. It seems, then, that as we fatigue our higher centers of control are lost first, leading to uncontrolled energy release and, finally, to full fatigue.

It is because our brains work this way, of course, that we have this type of behavior on fatiguing. Seizures are associated with areas of the brain that are inflamed. Edema is one of the features of inflammation. An area of the brain that is chronically inflamed, perhaps due to sleeping patterns, will be especially low in oxygen and sugar, and will possibly lose its self-control, eliciting a seizure.

In addition, some women have seizures a couple of days before their menstrual period. This is the same time that many women experience migraines. During this time the blood levels of estrogen, the female sex hormone, are elevated. One of the effects of estrogen is to increase fluid retention within the body, creating generalized edema, as we discussed for menstrual migraines. If a woman already has brain edema from sleeping too flat for too long, then this retained fluid may make the brain edema worse. This connection between menstruation and seizures shows the relationship between seizures and migraines, and between both of these conditions and brain edema.

Seizures and Migraines

Guess what condition is also known to *cause* seizures? That's right – migraines. In children especially, migraines can cause seizures, ataxia (abnormal muscular coordination), vomiting, stupor (a state of semi-consciousness), and delirium (a condition of temporary mental excitement and confusion, marked by hallucinations, delusions, anxiety, and incoherence). This connects migraines to seizures, in addition to other brain abnormalities.

And another cause of recurrent seizures is hypoglycemia, or low blood sugar. If the brain cannot get its sugar, it loses its control. Can you get sugar if the brain has edema? Only with difficulty. A person with brain congestion due to lying too flat for too long will have low sugar levels in the brain, which will be more or less exaggerated for any given area of brain, depending upon the brain circulation.

Seizures, then, may arise from the very same problem that causes migraines. How many people are told that they are epileptic, when they are simply congested in the brain? It could be many.

Looking at the Eyes

Let's shift the discussion to another part of the brain, but which few people realize is an extension of the brain itself. We are referring to the eyes. The venous drainage of the eyes is via the ophthalmic veins, which drain into the internal jugular vein, as is the case with most other veins of the brain. Arteries leading to the eye, the ophthalmic arteries, derive from the internal carotid artery, as is the case with most other arteries of the brain.

If the brain is excessively pressurized, then so are the eyes. What could this cause?

The eyeball is divided into two main chambers. The back chamber, in which resides the retina of the eye, is filled with a jelly like substance, called the vitreous body. The front part of the eye, which is around the colorful iris area, is filled with a watery substance, called the aqueous humor. The vitreous body forms 80% of the bulk of the eye and is fairly stable throughout one's lifetime. The aqueous humor, however, is constantly secreted and reabsorbed. It is very much like clear plasma and bathes the structures in the front of the eye, such as the iris, the outer surface of the lens, and the inside of the cornea. It is secreted by certain cells in the front chamber of the eye near the lens, called the ciliary process. The fluid then circulates around the lens and through the pupil, which is the hole in the iris, and creates an aqueous space that helps to hold out the cornea. The aqueous humor is important in light refraction and the creation of a clear image on the retina, which is located on the inside wall of the back of the eyeball, past the vitreous body.

Glaucoma

The aqueous humor must drain since it is constantly being secreted, and it does so through a venous sinus and then into nearby veins. It is known that obstruction of this drainage causes increased pressure within the eyeball. When obstructed, the chamber with aqueous humor is first pressurized. This pressure then affects the vitreous humor. The vitreous cannot compress in response to the pressure, so the pressure is further passed on to the retina and the blood vessels that feed it. This can create a problem. Unrelenting pressure on the retina cuts down on the blood vessels supplying the delicate retinal tissue. The purpose of the retina is to sense light and communicate that sensory information to the brain. The retina, in other words, is necessary for seeing. If the pressure in the eye impinges upon blood vessels that feed the retina, then the retina begins to deteriorate, along with one's sight. This condition is called glaucoma.

The term glaucoma refers to a group of eye diseases characterized by increased pressure within the eyeball. Glaucoma is caused by some failure in the reabsorption of aqueous humor from the front section of the eyeball. The cause is considered unknown, particularly in the slow, progressive form of the disease.

However, when you consider the possible cause of head pressure, and therefore of eye pressure, the mystery is solved.

Glaucoma and Head Pressure

Glaucoma is a disease of the elderly, which suggests that it may be the result of a lifelong, chronic process. What is happening is that chronic head congestion and pressure due to lying flat is inhibiting the drainage of the eyeball's aqueous humor. Without gravity, the only force promoting the drainage of the eyeball fluid is the pressure created by the cells secreting the fluid. If the venous drainage from the eye is hampered, however, as when lying down and losing the aid of gravity, this pressure created by cellular secretion can cause increased pressure within the eyeball itself. When vertical, however, gravity can help reduce the blood pressure in the veins and allow the aqueous humor to better drain. In addition, when lying down the pressure on the eyes is increased, as it is in the entire head, and this can increase the secretion of aqueous humor from the ciliary process. Therefore, lying down pressurizes the eyes by creating excess aqueous humor, and resists venous drainage from the head and eyes. Standing erect reduces aqueous formation and assists drainage from the eyes, reducing eye pressure.

Glaucoma researchers, to their credit, did not ignore gravity.[6] Glaucoma has been connected to migraines and head pressure. Studies have been made of the pressure changes in the eye that occur when you lie down and sit up. (See references) It was shown in many studies of this phenomenon that pressure in the eyes goes up considerably when you lie down. And the pressure goes down when you sit up. This is true for people with and without glaucoma.

One researcher, clearly fascinated with this gravity effect, actually tested eye pressure in people whom he had hang upside down. The pressure in the eyes hugely increased. What was his conclusion from this experiment? You would think that it would be that people with glaucoma should sleep with their heads elevated, to reduce eye pressure. But his conclusion was different. It was that people with glaucoma should not hang upside down! [7]

The Aging Brain

This example of glaucoma as a result of chronic head congestion and pressure brings up another disease of aging, one that threatens the very identity and lives of its victims. Its cause is also considered unknown. It is characterized by general deterioration of the brain. The brain's ventricles are enlarged. There is more cerebral spinal fluid, but less brain substance. It is what you would expect would happen to the brain after years of edema. Edema can cause pockets of deterioration within the brain, as tissue chronically deprived of nutrients and oxygen cannot properly function or heal, and ultimately breaks down. As the tissue deteriorates, fluid begins to fill in the spaces. All brain functions suffer. The highest brain functions will be the first to go, since, as with seizures, loss of control comes before loss of function. This leads to emotional outbursts, anxiety, and other psychological troubles. As the brain further suffers in its oxygen and nutrient depleted state, the brain loses progressively more functions, ultimately leaving the person in a depersonalized, vegetative state.

Can you name this disease? It is called presenile dementia, or Alzheimer's disease. We believe that Alzheimer's disease is the outcome of a lifetime of brain edema, and is related to the gravity and sleep position effect that causes migraines.

Alzheimer's Disease and Other Dementias

One form of dementia, called progressive hydrocephalic dementia, is similar in presentation to Alzheimer's disease and doctors try to differentiate between the two. This dementia is known to result from interference with the absorption of cerebral spinal fluid. The cause of this interference, however, is considered to be unknown, but we believe that it may be the same as for migraines. That is, reduced blood drainage from the brain due to lying flat can reduce the reabsorption of cerebral spinal fluid into the venous blood supply, increasing cerebral spinal fluid pressure. The cerebral ventricles are enlarged in this dementia, which is what you would expect from high pressure in the cerebral spinal fluid, and there is edema around the ventricles.

There is another dementia condition, called normal pressure hydrocephalus, in which the brain has extra cerebral spinal fluid and expanded ventricles, but normal cerebral spinal fluid pressure. It is known to be caused by an obstruction of or by resistance to the normal flow of cerebral spinal fluid, causing the fluid to build up in the brain. Why is the pressure not greater in this condition of excess brain fluid? It is because the fluid is simply filling in the spaces created by brain tissue deterioration. The deterioration may have been caused by chronic edema, as with Alzheimer's disease. Once the brain starts deteriorating, the fluid merely fills in the empty spaces. This condition also leads to difficulty walking, suggesting a possible connection with Parkinson's disease, as we will discuss below. In fact, Alzheimer's disease has been linked with Parkinson's disease, as well. And Parkinson's is known to lead to dementia.

Could it be that these various dementias – Alzheimer's disease, progressive hydrocephalic dementia, and normal pressure hydrocephalus — are simply different manifestations of the same problem of chronic brain edema from sleeping behavior? Might we simply be considering different dementia effects arising from the same lifestyle cause?

Rethinking Alzheimer's

Alzheimer's disease, like the other dementias mentioned, is known to be associated with brain edema. Edema is well recognized as a cause of tissue degeneration, since it leads to a lack of oxygen and sugar, effectively choking and starving the edematous tissue. Oxygen depletion by itself is enough to kill cells. Oxygen also is required to allow the cells to get energy from sugar. The cells cannot properly carry out their functions, repair themselves, secrete neurotransmitters, or grow when starved and choked of oxygen. Additionally, edema prevents the removal of waste products from the tissues. This means that the cells suffering from edema are sitting in their own waste, getting poisoned by their own products of metabolism. All cellular functions suffer as a result.

Some of the defining features of Alzheimer's disease are the presence in the brain of tangled nerve fibers and plaques, which are degenerated nerve endings. These observations, made during autopsies of Alzheimer's patients, have been thought to be the cause of the disease, although it is not known what causes the tangles and plaques. However, these tangles and plaques may be the effect of low oxygen levels, not the cause of the disease. All systems dysfunction when oxygen is low. Any unusual brain substance or function can be a product of cellular troubles resulting from low oxygen.

It has also been thought that aluminum can cause Alzheimer's, since autopsies have shown an excess of this metal in the brain. Others suggest that mercury, iron, calcium, zinc, selenium, and other elements may be accumulating in the brain, leading to Alzheimer's. Of course, this could also be an effect and not a cause. This is because the brain is normally protected against these elements by the blood-brain barrier. As we have explained, the tightness of cerebral arterioles and capillaries prevents many substances from crossing from the blood into the brain tissue. This protective mechanism is particularly effective against charged particles, such as metals, and is less effective against fatty substances, which have no charge. The metals suspected of causing Alzheimer's circulate in the blood in the charged state, preventing them from crossing the blood-brain barrier and entering the brain.

Why might they get into the Alzheimer's brain? The blood-brain barrier is only effective so long as its cells remain healthy. Deterioration of the cells lining brain arterioles and capillaries is a known outcome of brain edema. This means that brain edema will ultimately lead to vascular deterioration, further edema, and leakage of all sorts of substances into the brain, such as aluminum, or mercury, that would otherwise have been excluded by the blood-brain barrier. Studies have shown that the blood-brain barrier is defective in Alzheimer's patients. (See references)

Interestingly, anti-inflammatory drugs have been shown to reduce the incidence of migraines and Alzheimer's. Inflammation is an immune response to tissue damage. We usually think of inflammation when the body is fighting an infection. However, tissue repair is also under the supervision of the immune system, and involves inflammation. Edema is one of the central features of the inflammatory response. Its purpose is to provide fluid to help flush away cellular debris and other products of tissue restoration and repair.

A generalized inflammation of the brain is characteristic of Alzheimer's disease, and may be the product of cellular and tissue decay resulting from chronic edema and reduced brain perfusion. In other words, edema from lying too flat for too long causes tissue deterioration, which in turn causes an immune response to clean up and repair the tissue, which leads to more edema. Of course, this repair process cannot be successful if the brain continues to be congested because of one's sleeping behavior. Anti-inflammatory drugs have been shown to reduce the swelling in the brain and improve memory in Alzheimer's patients, as well as slow the progress of the disease. This suggests that brain edema is the problem that needs to be treated. All that we know of Alzheimer's, then, can be explained by brain edema. And the brain edema can be explained by the gravity/sleep effect.

Parkinson's Disease and Brain Hypertension

This brings us to another brain dysfunction that we will discuss in relation to increased head pressure. We will now consider the mechanical effect of expansion within the brain causing one brain area to impinge on adjacent areas.

This mechanical effect is apparent in brain tumors, when brain structures are literally pushed out of the way by the growing mass, leading to dysfunction in the shifted brain area. However, fluid pressure can also shift brain structures. Pressure in the ventricles, as seen in progressive hydrocephalic dementia, is known to impinge on the brain centers, or nuclei, that surround the ventricles, causing dementia. The brain does not like to be pushed aside. Pressure from pushing can cut down on circulation to that tissue, leading to edema, low oxygen, and deterioration. High brain pressure, then, can cause various disorders as a simple product of mechanical compression or shifting of brain tissue in response to the pressure.

This means that high blood pressure would be associated with various brain problems, since the hypertension would lead to increased brain pressure. Ventricles may or may not expand, depending upon the tissue pressure surrounding them. If centers of the brain become affected by this combination of edema and pressure, they can begin to malfunction and decay. One common condition that is known to result from this situation is Parkinson's disease.

The brain has certain neural tracts that act as "nerve cables" through which information is communicated, and several centers, or nuclei, which serve as processors and integrators of that information. The basal nuclei are key centers in the brain. They are small areas of brain tissue that surround the ventricles and are responsible for the planning, initiation, maintenance, and termination of movement. They monitor and mediate commands from the higher centers of the brain, and in general maintain muscle tone and control movement and balance. They influence all of our muscular activity. Diseases of these basal nuclei include dyskinesia, or difficulty in performing voluntary movements, and dystonias, or abnormal muscle tone. They also include Parkinson's disease.

Ventricular hypertension, or high pressure in the brain's ventricles, is caused by chronic brain congestion and pressure and can lead to edema around the ventricles. This means that structures surrounding the ventricles will suffer from edema, and these can include the basal nuclei and the tracts leading to and from them. Parkinson's is associated with hypertension, and can progress to dementia. The disease usually begins with the development of tremors, followed by a stiff, shuffling walk, trembling, and a fixed facial expression. Dementia is a late manifestation of the disease. There exists a muscular coordination problem, as with normal pressure hydrocephalus, which can be caused by brain edema. Indeed, the symptoms of Parkinson's can be explained by brain edema, particularly around the brain's ventricles, and affecting the basal nuclei, which are known to deteriorate in Parkinson's.

Stroke, seizure, glaucoma, Alzheimer's and Parkinson's may all thus be related to the same simple gravity/sleep effect that creates migraines.

Sinusitis and the Common Cold

If the brain has edema, then the rest of the head has edema, as well. Puffy eyes and congested sinuses can be an indication of face edema. If the sinus membranes are chronically edematous, creating sinusitis, then this can lead to tissue degeneration as happens to other tissues of the body suffering from edema. The integrity of the sinus membranes is essential for resisting the invasion of viruses and bacteria. Membranes starved of oxygen and nutrients due to edema, however, may not be able to repair and maintain their integrity, making infection more likely.

Edema in the sinuses also diminishes the activity of the immune system and creates a fluid environment ripe for the growth of disease-causing organisms. These factors add to the possibility of getting a sinus infection. This means that the common cold, which is caused by invading viruses, may be preventable by elevating the head while sleeping to minimize or eliminate sinus edema. This may also make it easier to breathe, allowing better oxygenation of the blood and greater overall vitality. Sinusitis has already been cured by head elevation.[8] Unfortunately, nobody has applied this knowledge to the common cold.

Peripheral Vascular Disease

Can there also be problems outside of the head due to brain congestion and pressure? One possibility relates to peripheral vascular disease.

In this set of diseases the blood supply to the legs and sometimes the arms is impaired. The cause may be within the blood vessels themselves. Atherosclerotic plaques, for example, cause the narrowing of the large and medium size arteries of the legs in a condition called arteriosclerosis obliterans, a type of peripheral vascular disease. Peripheral refers to structures away from the center of the body, such as the legs and arms. If these vessels narrow, then blood cannot be properly delivered to the limbs, and this results in oxygen depletion and starvation of those tissues. Gravity, of course, aids the blood going down the arteries to the limbs. However, the venous blood that needs to return to the heart is resisted by gravity, and this can cause edema in the limbs and further inhibit arterial delivery of blood. Remember that circulation requires that blood come in and be able to go out. You need both arterial supplies and venous drainage. The effect of gravity is well known in these vascular problems, and people realize that when they raise their legs or arms the swelling in them slowly goes down. The swelling is edema due to insufficient return of venous blood to the heart. However, if the arteries leading to the extremities are too narrow, then there will not be adequate supplies of oxygen and nutrients, or sufficient removal of cellular waste and carbon dioxide, resulting in ulcers and other signs of limb deterioration.

What does this have to do with the head?

In the carotid arteries of the neck are pressure receptors, as we have mentioned, which detect excessive pressure from the heart and provide a feedback to the heart to reduce the pressure. This mechanism is designed to regulate the blood pressure to the brain, preventing all the brain edema problems that we have been discussing. However, as the head receives the benefit from this carotid artery pressure safety mechanism, the rest of the body must also deal with reduced blood pressure. In other words, blood pressure goes down when we lie down, and this can affect the rest of the body, especially if there is already too little blood pressure in peripheral arteries due to some disease, such as arteriosclerosis obliterans. Excessive pressure in the head, then, can lead to too little pressure in the feet. Raising the bed and reducing this head pressure may help increase the pressure to the extremities.

Impotence

Peripheral vascular disease affects another limb besides the legs and arms. It also affects the penis. The mechanism we have just described of reduced blood flow to the limbs due to elevated head pressure can also lead to reduced genital perfusion, possibly causing a slow degeneration of penile function. This may be one cause of impotence.

In fact, vascular disease is a recognized cause of impotence, although the association between vascular disease and head elevation is a new connection we are making. Impotence, however, has many other recognized causes. Can head congestion lead to impotence by more than one mechanism? In other words, can the swelling of one head prevent the swelling of another?

Besides peripheral vascular disease, impotence is usually associated with brain or neurologic dysfunction. All forms of brain and neurologic dysfunction can be easily explained by edema of the brain, as we have shown. When the brain is edematous, its low oxygen and sugar levels prevent the proper functioning of various brain systems, including its nervous pathways and hormone secretions.

Erection and ejaculation require a concerted effort by all body systems to achieve optimal orgasm. A congested brain will not "fire" its nerves efficiently, interfering with the rhythm and tempo of the penis "firing". In addition, the pituitary gland in the brain is normally inhibited in its secretion of the hormone prolactin by chemical signals reaching the pituitary from the nearby brain control center, called the hypothalamus. Too much prolactin secretion is known to be a major cause of impotence. While it has never been understood why the control over prolactin secretion is lost in impotent men, we may now have the answer. A hypothalamus congested from a person sleeping too flat for too long may not be able to produce and secrete its inhibitory substances as well as a non-congested hypothalamus. This removes the normal controls over prolactin secretion, leading to hyperprolactinemia, or too high a prolactin level in the blood, and impotence.

Additionally, the brain must put out hormones to stimulate the testicles to secrete sex hormones. Low sex hormone levels cause impotence, too. A congested brain may only be capable of producing low levels of these stimulatory hormones, resulting in low testicular function and reduced male sex hormone production, leading to impotence.

However, there is a simpler way to see how brain congestion can lead to impotence. It follows from the fact that there are some men who experience migraines after having an orgasm, called an orgasmic headache. Why do some men get a headache after sex?

When you have an orgasm, the blood pressure rises to about the highest the body can stand. It already has to get pretty high for the penis to pressurize with blood and become erect. This is why men on high blood pressure medications typically become impotent. Their blood pressure gets too low. You need a good head of steam to get the penis going. However, as you build this steam for one head, the other head is also experiencing the increased blood pressure. Since the brain does not want to blow a blood vessel and develop a stroke, it follows that the brain, which ultimately controls penis function, would not allow an orgasm if that might cause the blood pressure to go too high. Impotence, then, may be the brain's way of preventing a stroke. The mechanism by which the brain creates the impotence may be through the prolactin mechanism just mentioned. Or it may be through some other interruption of the nervous pathways associated with the processes of erection or ejaculation.

Why are there orgasmic headaches? A brain that is already chronically congested will become even more so after weathering the increased blood pressure of the orgasm. Orgasms may thus further create brain edema in an already edematous head. In addition, the orgasm increases brain activity. This increases the brain's requirement for oxygen and sugar, which an edematous brain may already lack. The final outcome of the orgasm, then, can be a loss of fluid from one head, the gaining of fluid in the other head, and a splitting headache.

Women, of course, have orgasms, too, and this may create the same exceptionally high blood pressure peak that a congested brain does not want. It may, then, be that women who have difficulty reaching an orgasm may also be suffering from brain induced orgasm suppression. The clitoris is the anatomical equivalent of a penis, and has similar nervous supply. What's bad for the gander may also be bad for the goose.

We all knew that a headache is an excuse for not having sex. Now we may understand the reason why that is a good excuse.

Low Brain Pressure

You may be wondering why we have ignored cerebral hypotension, or low pressure in the brain. Could it be that standing for too long might drain the brain too greatly, so that it never has time to fully repressurize during horizontal time in bed? In other words, could there be chronic hypotension of the brain because of not enough lying flat or from lying flat for too short a period of time, the opposite of the effect of too much pressure by lying too flat for too long? The answer is maybe, but it seems to be rare.

The effect of hypotension on the brain is decreased buoyancy of the brain, causing it to descend when in the vertical position, exerting traction on structures at its apex and compression on structures at its base. This causes effects similar to a migraine, namely, headaches, nausea, vomiting, sensitivity to light, and a stiff neck. There could also be ringing in the ears and dizziness. These symptoms are thought to be due to gravity pulling on the brain without the resistance of the buoyant force of the cerebral spinal fluid. The cause of the fluid loss and consequent low pressure in the head is almost always leakage of cerebral spinal fluid after a spinal tap, or lumbar puncture. When a doctor inserts a needle into the lumbar space to check cerebral spinal fluid pressure, as described below, he may accidentally leave a hole through which cerebral spinal fluid can leak. Most patients with intracranial hypotension had just been through a spinal tap.

However, this is again the extreme case. Mild hypotension in the brain is typically managed by the brain's autoregulatory mechanisms. Brain arterioles dilate to increase blood supply and pressure. But let's assume that someone is vertical for too long and has low blood pressure. This would cause depletion in the brain of sugar and oxygen, since the fluid pressure would be too low. In a way, then, hypotension and hypertension of the brain can have similar effects on brain levels of oxygen and sugar. In hypertension this effect is caused by edema; in hypotension it is caused by low fluid volume. Both situations effectively reduce brain perfusion.

However, when we stand for too long, our heads get dizzy and we feel weak. We may even faint for lack of oxygen and sugar to the brain. So the body has a way of protecting itself from too little pressure. It makes you lie down, either voluntarily for a nap, or involuntarily, as when you faint.

The body, then, has a way to deal with low pressure in the brain. It makes us rest. We can ignore that message and take pep pills. Many people in today's frantic world don't feel that they have the time to rest, and complain of insufficient sleep. We have the ability to override our biological defense mechanisms. It's our culture that makes us do it. All other animals listen to their bodies' messages. Humans listen to their culture, even if it contradicts their bodies' messages.

This may be why some people experience migraines when getting too little sleep. Most report getting migraines from too much sleep, and wake up with the headache. If someone gets a migraine during the day, it may be from too low pressure in the brain. This can be aggravated by dehydration, since blood pressure is low when there is too little fluid. Either way, the migraine mechanism pressurizes the head. This may be to flush out an edematous brain, as we have described. Or it could be to pressurize an under-pressurized brain, as with hypotension.

Posture and Hypotensive Headaches

There is a very important fact known about the headaches caused by hypotension. The headaches are known to be affected by posture. The headache gets worse when standing up, and is relieved when lying down!

Imagine that! It is already known that low brain pressure and its associated headache are relieved by lying down, which increases head pressure. And it gets worse while standing, as gravity resists brain pressurizing and increases drainage. It is exactly the opposite of what happens when the head has too much pressure, as with migraines. Yet, this effect of posture has never been considered for migraines, which are known to be associated with increased brain pressure.

Most brain problems are caused by hypertension, not hypotension. This may be because it is easier to lie down than it is to get up. If we are forced to stay vertical we usually faint, which makes us horizontal. The brain needs to be repressurized or else it becomes dysfunctional. However, we need to listen to the alarm telling us when it's time to get up, that the re-pressurization is complete. In short, we need to listen to our bodies telling us what we need.

Gravity Effects Recognized in Medicine

Can medicine really have failed to connect gravity and sleep position to disease? Actually, it has made these connections in some cases, and has ignored them in others.

When you go to the doctor to tell you what you need for a neurological problem, such as migraines, the doctor may want to determine the pressure in the brain, or intracranial pressure. The doctor may not have ever considered the effect of gravity and sleep behavior on brain pressure. However, the doctor is trained to consider the effect of gravity when checking the fluid pressure in the brain.

To do this, the doctor performs what is called a lumbar puncture. In the lower back, near the waist, is the lumbar spine. In this area there is a region of the spinal cord where there is little cord and lots of cerebral spinal fluid. This area, of course, is in communication with the rest of the brain, so the fluid pressure in the lumbar spine should tell you the pressure in the brain. Naturally, the invasive act of sticking a needle into the spinal column is dangerous, and can create all sorts of problems, such as low brain pressure if the cerebral spinal fluid leaks out of the hole made by the needle. The procedure can also cause damage to nerves accidentally pierced by the needle, and brain infection caused by bacteria introduced by the procedure. Nevertheless, this is the typical method for determining cerebral spinal fluid pressure.

One thing a doctor performing the puncture must be certain of is that the head is on the same level as the lumbar spine. If the head is elevated on a pillow or incline table, it is known to reduce the head pressure relative to the lumbar spinal pressure, creating a false reading. If the head is lower than the lumbar spine, the head pressure goes up and the lumbar pressure goes down. Gravity is thus considered for spinal taps. Elevating the head clearly is known to reduce intracranial pressure.

Sudden Infant Death Syndrome (SIDS)

In all of the brain conditions mentioned thus far, researchers have seen a connection to edema, but have ignored the effect of gravity as modified by sleeping behavior as a causative factor.

However, the effect of head position during sleep as a cause of disease has been recognized in one particularly distressing condition. It is a problem that does not affect children or adults, but affects 1-12 month old infants. It is called Sudden Infant Death Syndrome, or SIDS. It is also called crib death. It results in the unexplained death of apparently healthy babies. Few clues to the disorder had been found in autopsies or by medical records. In most cases, the baby is found dead within a few hours of being put to sleep. The baby suddenly turns blue, becomes limp, and stops breathing. The infant does not cry out or struggle. It just stops functioning.

What clues are there as to the cause of SIDS? Death occurs within a few hours after the child is put to bed. Imagine a baby in bed. There are no pillows used for infants. Their heads are placed completely flat on the bed, which means that they can develop brain hypertension if left flat for too long. If this happens, the cerebral hypertension could lead to edema. If the parts of the brain responsible for breathing and blood pressure became too congested, it would interfere with their function. This could lead to brain dysfunction, failure, and death. Indeed, research has shown that babies who had died of SIDS had chronic brain hypertension. (See references)

Explaining the Risk Factors

Is there anything else to support this hypothesis? Premature babies are more likely to develop SIDS than full-term babies. Why may this be significant? Premature babies are more fragile than full-term babies are. Mothers are less likely to lift them and play with them, preferring to leave them alone in bed so as not to hurt them. This means the premature babies will be down for longer periods of time, and are more likely to develop brain edema. In addition, babies who are part of multiple births, such as twins or triplets, are at higher risk for SIDS. This makes sense, as well, since a mother has less time to spend lifting one baby when there are others who need attention and lifting, too.

By the way, this explains another fact, which is that breast feeding a baby lowers the risk for SIDS. This could be because a mother lifts her baby to her breast and cradles its head in an elevated position during nursing. Mothers who bottle-feed sometimes place the bottle in the crib alongside the baby, so the baby need not be lifted to feed. This, of course, means more down time for the bottle-fed baby.

Also, SIDS is much less likely to occur if the infant sleeps with his or her parents. This can be the result of two factors. First, the weight of the parents on the mattress creates a slight incline plane for the baby, elevating the baby's head. Second, when you sleep with a baby you often move the baby around, stimulating the circulation.

Another risk factor for SIDS includes smoking during pregnancy. Most likely, a woman who smokes while pregnant will also smoke after the baby is born. This increases the carbon monoxide in the air, causing a baby with an already edematous head to develop even lower oxygen levels in the brain, further depressing the brain's life support systems. SIDS deaths are also greater during the winter months. It is during this time that people close their windows to keep in the warm air. This also means that they keep the exhaust of their furnace, oven, and their own respiration inside the house. Carbon dioxide and carbon monoxide levels are higher inside the house than outside. This makes winter a more difficult time for infants with already compromised brain circulation.

Do you know what conclusion was finally reached as to the cause and prevention of SIDS? It was finally realized that babies who slept on their stomachs had the highest incidence of SIDS. It was reasoned that the impingement of the vertebral arteries supplying blood to the brain through the neck vertebrae might occur by the sideways positioning of the baby's head while placed on its stomach. This impingement reduces the blood supply to the brain, particularly the brain stem, which is responsible for breathing and basic life support functions. This creates low brain oxygen and can destroy the function of this part of the brain. A campaign to educate mothers not to put their babies to sleep on the stomach has helped reduce the incidence of crib death.

Adding the Element of Gravity

We think that this is only part of the answer. The baby may already have a congested, edematous brain due to spending much of the time horizontally. This makes impingement of the vertebral arteries by head turning more damaging. Without this added edema problem, you might expect that the carotid arteries could compensate for the impinged vertebral arteries, since they all connect around the Circle of Willis, as we have explained. Post-mortem autopsies did not find any abnormalities in these children's brains regarding blood vessel connections. However, this impingement of the vertebral arteries may be the last straw for an already congested and compromised brain.

The medical recommendation is for babies to be placed on their backs or sides for sleeping. This shows that gravity is still being ignored, since it reflects an interest in preventing vertebral artery impingement, not in preventing brain edema. It seems to us that infants should be placed on their backs, and that *their heads should be elevated*. Baby carriers, which place the baby in a slight hammock-like position, are probably better for the baby to sleep in than a flat crib. Sleeping with the baby, of course, is the best, since it allows a more natural interaction, stimulation, and movement of the baby.

Sleep Apnea

Altering sleep position as a disease treatment is also recognized in a sleep disorder called sleep apnea. This condition mostly affects middle-aged, overweight men, but anyone can have this problem. Hundreds of times each night, the tongue and throat drop back and obstruct the airways, stopping breathing for as long as 30-60 seconds each time! Of course, this prevents the brain and the rest of the body from getting oxygen, and it eventually elicits an emergency response from the brain to gasp for breath. People with sleep apnea, then, go through the night with repetitive cycles of breathing difficulty interrupted by gasping. The sufferer also typically has high blood pressure and heart problems.

An overweight person lying flat on his back will have difficulty breathing due to being overweight. It is difficult to lift a heavy ribcage to take a deep breath. Lying on the side would make rib cage expansion even more difficult, which is probably why these people lie on their backs. This difficulty in expanding the chest cavity results in less oxygen getting into the lungs, due to shallow breathing. This can make worse the already low oxygen levels in the brain due to lying flat. The fact that it can take 30-60 seconds for the brain respiratory centers to kick in and make the person gasp for air suggests a sluggishness in the brain's respiratory centers that may reflect chronic congestion.

One other response to oxygen deprivation, besides a gasp response, is an increase in blood pressure and pulse rate. The body needs oxygen. It can only get it through the blood. When the body is feeling desperate for oxygen, it tries to speed up the flow of blood to the brain and lungs to get whatever oxygen it can. Increased blood pressure and flow through the lungs maximizes the ability of the blood to get oxygen and discharge carbon dioxide. In other words, you would expect that a person who spends a third to a half of his or her life gasping for air to develop high blood pressure, which can lead to heart problems. Of course, being overweight can also cause high blood pressure and heart problems. However, the mechanism just mentioned may be an important additional factor.

How do you treat sleep apnea? One way is to lose weight, allowing the chest to better expand. Another way is to have a surgeon remove parts of the nose, throat, or jaw. Interestingly, another recognized way is to change sleep positions. Head elevation has been studied in treating sleep apnea, and it has been shown to work in eliminating the condition. (See references) Unfortunately, this is being ignored.

We suggest that the best position would be to elevate the head. If the head is elevated, gravity will not pull the tongue and soft palate back to obstruct the airways. The person should still stay on his back, since that makes chest expansion easiest.

There is one other interesting point about sleep apnea. In addition to the most common form of this condition, called obstructive (or positional) sleep apnea due to the obstruction of the airway by the tongue and throat, there is a less common form called central sleep apnea. In this form, no obstruction of the airway occurs. However, the diaphragm and chest muscles don't work properly because of a disturbance in the brain's regulation of breathing during sleep. This relates central sleep apnea to Sudden Infant Death Syndrome. It also suggests that the cause of the brain dysfunction could be due to edema, particularly of the brain stem, the part of the brain responsible for respiration. Of course, the cause of the edema is most likely the behavior of sleeping too flat for too long.

Obstructive and common sleep apneas, then, could be caused by the same lifestyle problem.

Finally, sleep apnea is commonly known to be associated with morning headache, intellectual deterioration, and reduced libido. This means that sleep apnea is connected to migraines, dementia, and impotence, which is exactly what you would expect for brain conditions arising from the same gravity/sleep effect.

Head Elevation Therapy

Some pediatricians recommend head elevation as a treatment for brain edema resulting from head trauma and Reyes' syndrome. Head trauma generates edema as part of the process of inflammation resulting from tissue damage. In Reyes' syndrome a virus attacks the brain and causes the blood vessels to leak, creating edema. To treat this edema, children are placed on a 15-30% incline plane to assist the brain in draining and to resist arterial pressure, just as we have described for migraines. It is even suggested that the children be placed on their backs and not on their sides or stomachs, since turning the head to the side can impinge the jugular veins in the neck.

In other words, the very same mechanism we have been proposing and have tested for migraines has already been in use by some pediatricians to do exactly what we claim it can do. While this treatment is not universally applied in medicine, the effect of head elevation on intracranial pressure has been measured, quantified, and established as helpful.

In addition, head elevation is standard procedure after brain surgery to relieve edema. It is also sometimes used to treat stroke.

Head elevation, as you can see, is nothing new to medicine. What we have done is apply a recognized therapy for brain edema to the prevention and treatment of other diseases associated with brain edema. Why this safe, free, effective way to treat and prevent brain edema has not been publicized for general practice is a question we will further address in the final chapter.

Individual Responses to Excessive Head Pressure

If all of these conditions can be explained by increased head pressure, then why is it that some people will manifest the problem by a seizure, others by a stroke, others by getting migraines, and still others by developing Alzheimer's disease, Parkinson's, or sleep apnea? The answer is that we are all unique in structure and function.

It is known that the arterial traffic circle in the brain, the Circle of Willis, has different connections in different people, altering the ability for one artery to supply blood to another artery. Blood vessels have the ability to connect with other blood vessels to create alternate pathways. These connections are called anastomoses. The brain has anastomoses between its arteries, arterioles, and veins. But every brain has its own particular connections. This means that obstruction of one particular brain blood vessel may be compensated for by an anastomosis in one person's brain better than in another person's brain.

In addition, the ventricles of the brain are connected to one another through very thin tube-like channels. The thinness of these channels can affect how well the cerebral spinal fluid can flow throughout the brain. Some people may have been born with particularly narrow channels, leading to a particular manifestation of excessive head pressure.

Then there is the effect of sleeping. Gravity works on us even when we are lying down, making the part of the head that is highest have less pressure than the part of the head that is lowest. Certain blood vessels in the neck can be impinged upon by sleep position, as with SIDS. Whether you sleep on your right or left side, or on your back or stomach, will make a difference to the brain. In addition, a tight neck can have a major influence on brain circulation. How tight the neck is and which blood vessels are impinged by that tightness is another variable that may affect how that brain congestion may manifest in any given person. We will discuss these important considerations in the next chapter.

The Migraine Connection

The diseases we have discussed, including migraines, may have more than one cause. Undoubtedly, there are constitutional, or genetic, predispositions to many of them, as well as environmental conditions that promote them. What we have tried to show is that the cultural issue of sleep position and its relationship to the effect of gravity is the primary issue creating these problems, and will further exacerbate all brain conditions. This new theory can also connect various brain conditions that, until now, have been considered separate entities with an unrelated or unknown cause.

There are thousands of articles connecting migraines to the following medical conditions: brain edema; brain ischemia; cerebral hypoperfusion (poor circulation); intracranial swelling; cerebral spinal fluid pleocytosis (white blood cells in the fluid, a result of edema);

progressive cerebellar ataxia (loss of muscular coordination); increased cerebral spinal fluid pressure; cerebral infarcts (areas of damaged tissue due to lack of circulation); cerebral ischemic accidents (strokes); hypoxic cerebral vasodilation (vasodilation due to low oxygen); edema of the cerebral cortex; hydrocephalus (cerebral spinal fluid accumulation in the ventricles of the brain or around the outside of the brain); glaucoma; ischemic stroke; epilepsy; Pre-Menstrual Syndrome; chronic intracranial pressure; sleep apnea; hypoglycemia; diabetes; high altitude sickness; and impotence.

These are some of the many pieces of the puzzle. It makes it seem as though these were completely separate conditions. However, once you add the missing pieces of gravity and sleep, it allows you to see a common mechanism for them all.

Does this mean that migraines are a diseased condition, or a survival mechanism? Brain stagnation, edema, and pressure cannot be healthy for you. The same problem, lying too flat for too long, that leads to a migraine response may also cause other problems. However, migraines don't cause these other problems. They may just be a reaction to the problem of edema. It is similar to a fever, which is a response to an infection and not the cause of the infection. The fever is not a symptom of a disease, but a healthy mechanism for curing it. Likewise, excessive brain pressure and edema is a disease-causing condition, and migraines may simply be a healthy mechanism to correct it.

Are Migraines Protective?

You would think that, if migraines were indeed protective, then people who have migraines may be better off than others who, for some reason, may have high intracranial pressure yet do not get migraines. There should be some advantages to migraines, just as we would assume that there should be some advantages to people who get a fever early on in the infection, instead of waiting for the infection to do more damage.

Indeed, this is the case. People with migraines have lower incidence of cerebrovascular and ischemic heart disease than the non-migrainous public. (See references) Why would this be the case? Cerebrovascular disease relates to the brain's blood vessels. Perhaps the migraine response spares the brain's blood vessels of the ravages of chronic, unchecked edema, which could cause the vessels to deteriorate. Ischemic heart disease means too little blood to the heart. Without migraines, a chronically congested brain in the horizontal position would reduce blood pressure as much as it could to survive. To do this the heart has to be slowed down. This is accomplished with hormones and nervous signals from the brain and carotid arteries, lowering heart function and blood delivery to the heart itself. A migraine response, however, may solve the brain's congestion problem without excessively lowering blood pressure and effecting the heart's circulation.

Finally, researchers have found that the abrupt cessation of migraines was sometimes one of the earliest indications of degeneration of the brain. (See references) This may indicate two possibilities. It may mean that degeneration hampers the ability of the brain to mount a migraine response, suggesting that the migraine response is a healthy function that is lost upon degeneration. (If it were itself a degenerative process, you would expect that it would increase upon brain degeneration.) Also, it may mean that migraines help prevent degeneration, and when the brain no longer has migraines, degeneration sets in.

The Migraine Advantage?

If migraines are protective, then what happens to people who don't get them? Why do only some people with brain edema get a migraine response? It may be that a threshold of edema must be reached before a migraine response is elicited. People with mild to moderate brain edema may not exceed this threshold, keeping their brains continually congested. A migraine may require a bit more edema to elicit a flushing response. However, once this flushing occurs, the brain may return to a much lower state of congestion than that of a brain that has not had a migraine. Some people report feeling a heightened sense of well being after a migraine. (See references) This may be why. For those who remain chronically congested, the brain may proceed down a path of progressive deterioration, leading to other congestive brain dysfunctions.

Several other researchers have speculated that migraines may be protective, and may even promote survival, as we mentioned. There is nothing new under the moon, either. Yet, this is a rare thought, virtually lost among the mountains of research on migraines and the drugs that may treat it. It was a thought that was clearly abandoned, since it is no more than wild conjecture without a mechanism to explain how migraines can be advantageous. For this you need to think of the whole person, gravity, and how our culture trains us to sleep.

What is really needed is a science of sleep that considers the effect of gravity and body position on the structure and function of the body. We shall now begin to explore this new science, and see what it tells us about the healthiest way to sleep.

6

It's All In Your Bed

What exactly is sleep?

People have been asking this question ever since there have been people. And they still have no clue to its answer.

All we can really say about sleep is that it is one of our experiences, a part of our reality. We don't really know what life is, either. These are philosophical, perhaps even theological, questions that have been debated for millennia. If we can't even agree on what life is, then how can we begin to understand sleep?

Measuring Sleep

In the absence of an answer to these questions, scientists offer some measurements. It is easier to measure something than it is to know what it is that you are measuring. So when it comes to sleep, scientists use a machine that detects electrical waves produced by the brain, creating an electroencephalogram, or EEG. The brain seems to produce different EEG tracings made by the machine, depending on the brain's activity at the time. Sleep has its own type of EEG tracing, and scientists who study sleep spend sleepless nights trying to differentiate between subtle changes in EEG tracings and how that might relate to various stages of sleep. Any sleep book will go into the elaborate scheme that they have developed. Of course, it still does not tell you what sleep is.

One older theory[9] attributes sleep to changes in cerebral circulation. It was thought that congestion and retarded movement of blood in the brain's vessels, particularly the veins, or from a diminished flow of arterial blood to the brain, leads to sleep. It seems that brain circulation during sleep has been an issue considered before now. However, ignoring the relationship between sleep position and gravity, this theory confuses the effect — diminished brain circulation and consequent congestion, with the cause — lying down flat to sleep. It is sleep that congests the brain, not congestion that leads to sleep.

What sleep really "is", in the ultimate metaphysical sense, is impossible to answer with certainty. All of our conclusions are conditioned upon our experience, which is always limited, particularly when it comes to the subject of sleep. Yet, we must live despite our uncertainty over exactly what life is. And we must sleep with the same uncertainty about that activity. Actually, the best question to ask is not what sleep is, but rather how does sleep affect us. That is all that really counts.

Understanding Sleep

To understand the roles that sleep serves in our lives we must consider the circumstances and features of our lives. This is a cultural issue, not a biological one, and it has absolutely nothing to do with EEG's. However, before we discuss the role of sleep in our modern, western society, let's imagine ourselves living in a more natural, primitive state. What role might sleep have in our primitive lives? This query may shed light on how nature "intended" humans to sleep.

Primitive Sleep Research

By "primitive" we mean a culture of people living close with nature, without the material conveniences and contraptions of "civilized" life, such as housing, bedrooms, and king sized beds. Imagine, for example, a tribe of forest-dwelling Indians. These people would certainly value sleep for its dreams and mystical insights. The dream world can feel as real and important to us as our awake world, if our culture sanctions and promotes such a view. If you valued dreams, your sleep would be a special and important time. However, to enjoy that time you must not feel as though you might be attacked at any moment. In a way, sleep makes you vulnerable. It is a luxury to be able to totally lose consciousness of this "awake" world and enter the dream world.

If times were more dangerous, you would imagine that sleeping might be considered something you needed to do, but it must wait for the appropriate, safe time. Warriors, for example, may have their moments of dream world insights and prophecies. But they cannot insist on getting their full 8-10 hours per night. At times of aggression, they may have to go days without sleep, or catch a short nap when they can and if they absolutely needed it.

Naturally, most of the time as a primitive person you would be between these two extremes. There would be times of relative peace, when sleep would serve as an entertaining, prophetic, or simply otherwise enjoyable personal time. However, you would never be sure when that peace might be broken, either by human or animal attack. Sleep, then, must also have its practical side. It is something that you need to do, but it should not get in the way of other life functions.

This raises a practical question. Given the fact that you may have to jump up in the middle of sleeping in order to respond to an intruder, how do you think you should sleep?

As a primitive person, you cannot consult a magazine or health care book for an answer, so you have to just use your own reasoning. First, you notice that your ears are on opposite sides of your head.

Hearing is an especially important sense in the dark of night. We hear things moving before we see them, particularly when our eyes are closed. So you reason that you should keep your ears open. This means that you would not want to be sleeping on your side, since this would limit your hearing. You would be able to hear with the up ear, but it would not be stereo, as it is with two ears. The stereo effect allows you to locate the source of a sound, just as having two eyes allows you to have depth perception and better locate a visual object in space. One ear may hear the sound, but that may not let you know exactly from where the sound originated. So you conclude that you probably should sleep either on your back or your stomach, to keep your ears open.

You then perform a simple, primitive experiment on yourself and try sleeping on your stomach. Soon you realize that there is a slight problem. You can hear things just fine. But you cannot see what you are hearing since your eyes are facing downward. It also feels uncomfortable to have your entire head leaning on your nose. It makes breathing difficult and hurts your neck. So the next night you perform another experiment and sleep flat on your back. This time you can breathe clearly, which you realize is useful for identifying intruders coming from up wind. Yet, there is still a problem. When your ears detect a sound you can now open your eyes to see what's there. But you can only look straight up.

A few days later, while sleeping flat on your back, you discover another problem with your sleeping position. In the middle of the star lit night you detect the sound of something moving in the bushes nearby. Your anxious mind responds to the sound, since you cannot afford to be a heavy sleeper, and you open your eyes and quickly jump to your feet anticipating trouble. Fortunately, it's only your dog. Your mind tells you that it's not an emergency, and that you can relax. But your heart starts pounding and you feel dizzy, making you sit down. Since you haven't any medical books, you don't realize that you were experiencing orthostatic hypotension, or low blood pressure upon standing. All you know as a primitive person is that when you get up too fast from a flat position it makes you dizzy and sick to your stomach for a while. Of course, you have no idea about gravity and its effect on your brain when you are lying down compared to when you are standing up. So you scratch your head in bewilderment and feel disappointed that your sleeping arrangement is not yet perfect.

Migraines of Antiquity

Years later you start to get headaches. They are very painful, and as a primitive person you come up with the best answer that your culture can muster to explain your pain – you're possessed by evil spirits. You sacrifice a chicken to the appropriate deity and hope for no more of this pain. But no luck. It becomes a recurrent punishment in your life. You feel you have done something for which the gods are making you pay. So you plead and cry to the gods for your salvation. Nothing works. Defeated and disgusted with life, you go to the medicine man for help. He has no idea what is causing your headaches, either. However, he does a special surgical procedure that he is willing to try on you. He says that there have been some reports of its success, but there are no guarantees. Feeling desperate, you agree. The next time you have your headache you go to the medicine man. He places your head down on a soft bed of grass. Some large men approach and lean their weight on your body, making it impossible for you to move. And he slowly, but effectively, begins to bore a hole through your skull. "This will let out the evil spirits", he explains.

Anthropologists have discovered actual ancient human skulls with holes bored into them. It is assumed that this was one form of migraine treatment. It's too bad that the hammock had not yet been developed in that primitive culture. This would allow the head to be above the heart, preventing over-pressurization, and still allow the feet to drain, since they, too, are slightly elevated in a hammock. Many primitive people, and some other primates, such as orangutans, sleep in hammocks. They probably never get migraines.

91

Modern Sleep Science

Most people in today's "modern" cultures sleep in beds and not in hammocks. Since modern civilization has developed the sciences of physiology and anatomy to better understand the working of our bodies, surely we can use that basic information to develop a science of sleep. What, then, are the health consequences of various sleep positions, and what is the healthiest way to sleep?

Let me caution the reader to maintain an open mind when considering these factors. We all feel attached to our sleeping behavior. It is part of our private, unself-conscious time. It's our time to feel that we are back in the womb, warm, safe, and free from the problems of the world. Given this personal, idealized view of sleep, we resist thinking about changing sleeping patterns. Hopefully, our desire for health is greater than our attachment to a sleeping position.

Human Anatomy and Sleep

That said, let's consider the anatomy of the human body in its asymmetry. If you look at a person facing you, you will notice a plane of symmetry straight down the middle, from the top of the head through the pelvis. Most of the body consists of paired structures, such as two arms, two ears, two legs, and two eyes. But inside the body organs are not necessarily arranged along this midline. And paired organs are not necessarily the same size.

For example, we have two lungs, but the right lung is larger than the left lung. The heart is unpaired, and it lies slightly to the left of the midline. This is why the left lung is smaller than the right lung. It accommodates the heart.

As we proceed down the body we come to the abdomen. Here we find one stomach, and it is skewed to the left. All the way on the left of the stomach is the spleen, which stores blood as part of its function. To the right of the stomach is the liver, a huge and heavy organ located mostly to the right of the midline. Connected to the liver is the gallbladder. Beneath the stomach is the pancreas, an important hormone-producing and digestive organ. It is mostly to the right of the midline. Further down, past asymmetrical folds of intestine, there is the appendix, on the lower right side of the abdomen. The large intestine, or colon, ascends the abdomen from the area of the appendix, first going to the liver as it rises up the right side of the body, then taking a left turn to go beneath the liver and stomach towards the spleen on the left side, and then descending the left side, where it makes an "S" shaped bend as it goes into the lower pelvis and exits the body along the midline, at the anus. The largest section of the colon, then, is on the left side, particularly the part that fills with waste in preparation for later elimination.

Then there are the lymph nodes, which are asymmetrically scattered throughout the body, although there is some symmetry to the lymphatic system, as well. Lymph nodes in the groin and the armpits are relatively symmetrically arranged. There are other organs and structures that we have not discussed that have some asymmetries, but the major ones have been mentioned. Now, what does this have to do with sleep position?

The Problems of Side Sleeping

If you sleep on the side, organs on that side will be down relative to organs on the other side. Gravity will draw the top organs downward compressing the organs underneath. For example, let's say you sleep on your right side. This means that your left side is up. This allows your heart to have more room as it presses down on the right lung. The left lung will inflate easier than the pressed right lung. The left lung is smaller than the right, as we mentioned, which may mean that you cannot breathe as easily as if you were on your left side, with your right, larger lung in the up position.

Right side sleeping will also compress the liver and appendix. Appendicitis is thought to occur when digestive material gets lodged in the appendix, leading to infection. Leaning on the appendix as one sleeps on the right side, night after night, for hours each time, may provide a mechanism for appendix congestion and the development of appendicitis. The liver must also bear the weight of the stomach when lying on the right side. This might interfere with proper liver and gallbladder function, since a compressed organ does not have proper blood and lymph fluid circulation. It may also interfere with the return of blood from the intestines, since this blood first comes through the liver for processing of the newly absorbed digestive products. Liver compression may impede this blood flow, possibly causing a back up of blood in the intestines, leading to elevated fluid pressure and tissue edema, which would interfere with the entire digestive process.

If you sleep on the left side, then the heart will be in the down position, and the right lung will have dominance over the left lung. Pressure on the heart may interfere with proper cardiac function. Further down, the spleen will be compressed since it is on the left side. Given the fact that the spleen stores blood, compression may limit this storage capacity, increasing blood volume and raising blood pressure while on the left side. In addition, pressure on the colon, particularly the part that is filled with compacting waste material, may interfere with bowel function, as the small intestines lean into the "S" part of the large intestine while a person is on their left side.

This brief analysis is not meant to be exhaustive. Indeed, we hope that considerations such as these become part of a new field of sleep physiology. However, it does illustrate the significance of sleep posture on internal organ position and function.

Arms and Legs

Now to the more obvious issue of our limbs. Have you ever awakened from sleep to be shocked by a numb, cold, lifeless arm? All of us have experienced this at one time or another. Of course, it is caused by leaning on the arm while sleeping. The weight of the body presses on the poor limb, cutting off the blood supply. Soon, the nerves, starved of oxygen, lose their ability to function.

The entire limb starts to cool, since cells within the limb cannot produce their own heat due to lack of oxygen, and warm blood from the rest of the body cannot enter the compressed limb. Once the compression ends, however, the circulation can flush out the stagnant, deoxygenated blood, replacing it with fresh, oxygenated fluid. The nerves tingle as they recover their ability to respond to sensation. Soon, all you have left of the experience may be muscle tightness. Of course, this is the extreme scenario of limb compression. Mild compression may still impair circulation, but not enough to fully numb the limb.

What happens if you sleep on your arm every night, for hours each time? Chronic, recurrent compression of parts of the body may ultimately lead to dysfunction. If you spend one third of your lifetime compressing your left arm or hand, for example, would it be a surprise if you develop neuritis in the arm, or arthritis in that shoulder, elbow, or hand? Would it be a surprise if you had constantly tight and painful muscles in that arm? Compression prevents proper circulation. You cannot expect to have a healthy limb if you are limiting its circulation 8 out of every 24 hours, day after day, year after year.

Carpel Tunnel Syndrome

People who sleep on their hands may develop carpal tunnel syndrome. This tightness of the wrist is considered a "compression injury". Yet, no mention is ever made as to the cause of the compression. One erroneous solution told to the public is to wear an elastic, compression bandage around the wrist to stabilize the joint. It should seem strange to any thinking person to use a compression bandage to treat a compression injury. Why it is ever recommended is a mystery. Of course, if it doesn't work, there's the old standby — surgery.

The Compressed Breast and Pain, Cysts, and Cancer

Women who lie on their sides will be leaning on a breast, which may impair breast circulation. We have shown in our research into fibrocystic breast disease and breast cancer that compression from bras hampers the circulation in the breast, leading to toxin accumulation and edema, and resulting in disease. (See our book, *Dressed To Kill*) Sleeping on the side can lead to breast compression and limit the circulation, as well. Some women only remove their bras for sleep. If they then sleep on their sides, the down breast will not benefit from its brief reprieve from constriction. This is one reason why many women get breast cancer in one breast instead of in both at the same time.

Obviously, stomach sleeping will make matters worse for breast compression. As with side sleepers, stomach sleepers turn their heads to one side. This orients the body to that side, as well, making the breast on that side slightly less compressed than the other. Again, this asymmetric compression may help account for the asymmetry of breast disease. (Another factor is that bras are manufactured with both cups the same size, while nature does not necessarily manufacture women's breasts the same way. The larger breast will therefore be more constricted by the bra than the other breast.)

Penis Compression and Impotence

We know that crossing one leg over the other is bad for you, since the circulation to the legs will be impaired. Sleeping on the side effectively crosses one leg over the other. If you are a man, this may cause compression of more than the legs. If the testicles are compressed, then they will not receive an adequate blood supply or be allowed proper blood drainage, which may lead to testicular edema. This can interfere with sperm production and sex hormone production. This means that infertility may result from testicular compression due to side sleeping. And if the sex hormones production is reduced, this can lead to impotence. (We discussed impotence in chapter 5 as arising from brain edema.)

In addition, compression of the penis makes it bend to the side, as happens with the nose from side sleeping. If this compression can change the curvature of the penis, it can certainly alter the function of the penis. No organ likes to be bent and smashed for 6-12 hours daily, day after day, year after year. In addition, tight underwear continually smashes down the penis. A penis abused in this way may become incapable of proper erection and ejaculation. Impotence, like breast disease, may thus be another type of compression injury.

Of course, all these compressions are uncomfortable to us, even in our sleep. This is why people frequently toss and turn in bed. The body does not want to be compressed at one spot for long, so your brain makes you flip back and forth to aid the circulation and offer relief to the compressed area. This may make sleep less relaxing and comfortable. But if a person has a habit of sleeping on one side, he may resist his body's messages to turn. Some people get into their favorite sleeping position, perhaps curled up on the left or right side, the covers snugly tucked against the neck or over the back of the head, and they stay that way for 8 or more hours until morning. It's hard for the brain to deal with people like this.

Trigeminal Neuralgia

Some side sleepers may also complain about pain in the temples, jaw, or forehead, which is the distribution of a nerve in the face called the trigeminal nerve. The condition is called trigeminal neuralgia, which means severe pain along the course of the trigeminal nerve. This nerve, also called the fifth cranial nerve, originates in the brain and exits a hole in the skull to supply the face. It has been hypothesized that compression of the nerve by arteries lying near it in the brain can cause the neuralgia. Why arteries should suddenly compress the nerve is not mentioned. Of course, if you consider this a result of lying flat, then the picture is clearer. Pressure builds in the brain arteries in the absence of a gravity resistance, causing the arteries to bulge, thereby making them compress nerves near them. Arteries and nerves frequently travel close together.

On the other hand, one interesting aspect of trigeminal neuralgia is that it rarely occurs at night. This makes it seem less a sleep related disorder, since you would assume that sleep disorders only affect you when you are sleeping. However, remember that numb arm you slept on? It began to tingle and hurt once the blood supply returned to the limb and reactivated the nerves, which happened after you rolled over and got off the limb.

Keeping this in mind, we can propose another mechanism for trigeminal neuralgia.

If you sleep on your side, you will be compressing your jaw, temple and forehead for many hours each night. Sometimes you can hear your pulse while lying on your side, as the weight of your head compresses arteries near the ear. This area of the face is the distribution pathway of the trigeminal nerve. Compression reduces the circulation in the face just as it does in the arm, leading to nerve inactivation. Nerves don't like when you do this, and when you finally stop pressing on them they let you know their displeasure by tingling and giving you pain. The pain of trigeminal neuralgia usually lasts only seconds, just like the pain of a nerve trying to recover from compression. A head lying on its side is heavy, especially from the point of view of the trigeminal nerve being pressed upon. Of course, if the sleep pattern is not changed, the pain will return.

The cause of trigeminal neuralgia, then, could be excessive head pressure, distending the brain arteries to the point of their impingement on adjacent nerves. And it could be the direct result of mechanical pressure of the head onto the nerve due to side sleeping.

More Problems With Side Sleeping

There is another problem to side sleeping. If you sleep on your left side, then the left side of your brain may be more congested than the right side. As we have mentioned, the right side of the brain controls the left side of the body, and vice versa. So a right-handed person sleeping on their left side may experience some reduction in strength and function in their right arm, since their left brain is congested. Of course, since he is sleeping on his left arm, this arm will also experience a loss of strength and function, so it may feel equally bad in both arms. The same goes, of course, for lefties who sleep on their right side. Should a lefty sleep on his left side and a righty sleep on his right? It won't help. The stronger arm will be compressed, making it weaker, and the weaker arm will have its brain centers congested, making it weaker still.

Front Sleeping

If side sleeping is problematic, then how should we sleep? The answer cannot be sleeping on our front side. All the soft structures of the body are on the front surface. The rib cage expands and contracts using the breastbone, or sternum, as a hinge. That is, when we breathe deeply the ribs open up from the front of the body, as opposed to on the back where the ribs meet the backbone. Rib expansion is important since it allows you to breathe more deeply. When you breathe the chest cavity volume expands as the ribs lift and the diaphragm pulls downward, creating lower pressure in the chest cavity. This sucks air into the lungs. It also sucks blood from the abdomen up to the heart, and from the brain down to the heart. Breathing is known to affect general circulation in this way, but is not as effective as gravity in draining the brain. However, when we are lying down, and gravity is not working as a drain, breathing is the best mechanism we have. And deep breathing, which we all occasionally do when sleeping, creates better drainage than shallow breathing.

One specialized form of deep breathing is the yawn. Why do we yawn when fatigued? A yawn is a slow, sustained deep breath, creating several seconds of negative pressure in the chest. This returns blood from the body and head to the heart. It also creates a negative pressure within the lungs, making the lungs fill with air and blood, facilitating blood oxygenation and cleansing of carbon dioxide. This is why we yawn when fatigued. The brain drainage and circulation are increased and the blood gets oxygenated, further stimulating and supporting the functions of the brain.

If you lie on your side the chest can only partially operate as a brain drainage mechanism and blood oxygenator, since the down side of the chest cannot expand as easily as the up side. If you sleep on your chest, then this expansion is extremely limited. You cannot breathe deeply lying on your chest.

In addition, it is not easy to breathe with your nose flattened into the bed. So front sleepers typically turn their heads to one side, which allows for breathing but creates tight neck muscles and chiropractor appointments. This position can also possibly compress the vertebral arteries leading up the spine to the brain, as happens with SIDS, lowering brain perfusion. And it may compress the veins leading down from the brain. The facial compression for a stomach sleeper will also be greater than that for a side sleeper. There will probably be the telltale signs of a bent nose, puffy eyes, wrinkles, and sinus congestion.

Sleeping on the front also places pressure on the bladder, since this organ is near the surface of the front of the body, beneath the belly button. This means more trips to the bathroom and less sound sleep, since a compressed bladder will feel full sooner than a non-compressed bladder.

The Advantages of Back Sleeping

It seems that the best way to sleep is on the back. First, there is more surface area for you to lean the weight of your body upon, since the back of the body is wider than the sides. The sides have less than half as much surface area as the back, making the pressure on the side over twice that as when lying on the back. Further, the back of the chest cavity and abdomen is mostly composed of bone and muscle, which are heavy. If you sleep on the front, the internal organs must bear the weight of the back as it presses on them. When you sleep on your back, the lighter organs are pressing on the inside of the back, a much more favorable situation. The bladder can have more room and time to fill, and the colon will not have its packaging of waste material hampered by compression. In addition, men's genital organs and women's breasts will be spared hours of compression, affording better circulation and tissue health.

As we have said, the vertebral arteries supplying the brain are protected by the vertebral column from pressure while on the back. Sleeping on the side exposes the carotid arteries in the neck, as well as the neck veins, to possible impingement, since they do not have the benefit of a bony encasement to protect them. Back sleeping, therefore, minimizes the chance of vascular impingement during sleeping.

Not everyone is comfortable on their backs for sleeping, despite these considerations. I have always been able to sleep that way. However, Soma has tried over the years to be a back sleeper, but has failed. That is, until we elevated the head of our bed. Now she finds it more comfortable than any other position. We have now moved from the bed into a loveseat double-recliner. We cannot imagine sleeping any other way again. Regular beds seem too flat to us anymore.

It was from personal experience that we first began to think about these issues. Soma had always had sinus congestion and puffy eyes for as long as she could remember. And each month, at about the time of her menstrual period, she would get a headache. In fact, the headache always told her when her period was coming. Within months of raising our bed, however, she lost the morning stuffiness and her eyes were significantly less baggy. And her headaches disappeared. Now she needs a calendar to guess when her period is coming. (Her breasts used to get tender when her period was coming, too. But getting rid of her bra eliminated that problem, ending the constriction that was creating breast edema and the associated tenderness.)

The effect of sleeping one way for decades, however, will not be completely erased by head elevation. Soma still feels that the side of her face that she had habitually slept on is always more congested and tight-feeling than the other side of her face. Her nose bends slightly to the side because of the facial compression. And you can even see how side sleeping pushed her teeth out of proper alignment. But the body does heal, even if her teeth will not change their alignment and her nose will not straighten. She says her memory has improved since elevating her head. She can now recall names of people much more easily than when she had been sleeping flat. Her scalp is less tight and swollen. And she has more energy and a clearer mind than she can remember having since her youth. She even now feels as though she needs less sleep. In short, she looks and feels younger.

Head Elevation and Heart Function

Most people do not sleep on their backs. When you lie flat on your back in bed, your head will be almost at the same level as your heart. Once you become used to sleeping with your head elevated, as we now are, and you again try lying flat on your back, you can feel the pressure immediately building in your head. The external jugular vein, which returns blood from the head, will visibly pop up in the neck, as the blood from the head helplessly pools without the aid of gravity to return it to the heart.

Doctors assess the degree of heart failure in a patient by examining these distended neck veins. The patient lies flat on his back on the examination table. The table has a hinge in the middle allowing the top half of the table to be lifted. The lack of gravity draining the blood from the head to the heart causes the neck veins to pop up full of blood. The doctor lifts the table, slowly increasing the inclination of the patient's head. This increases the effect of gravity on the blood in the neck. A poorly pumping heart creates a worse backing-up of blood in the veins, as the blood waits for the heart to suck it in. This means that more gravity and higher head elevation are needed to drain the brain when the heart is not working at its best. At a certain elevation of the head, the swelling in the neck veins disappears. This indicates that the blood is now flowing to the heart. The worse the heart is working, the higher this level of inclination needs to be for the veins to disappear.

Of course, this assessment of heart failure by measuring the degree of head elevation needed to drain the neck veins should have led intelligent physicians to recommend head elevation for brain drainage regardless of heart failure. We all need the head elevated some degree for the neck veins to drain properly. Heart failure simply requires more elevation, say 45-degrees instead of 30-degrees. If we all require some elevation, why aren't we all told to sleep slightly elevated? We will try to answer this question in the next chapter. (By the way, heart failure patients are told to elevate their beds, but not for their brains. It's to assist lung drainage, preventing pulmonary (lung) edema.)

Flat Beds

Unfortunately, beds are designed to be flat. At one time mattresses were stuffed with straw, wool, cotton, or feathers, all of which are compressible. The body would make an impression in the mattress. Since the head is lighter than the torso, the impression in the mattress would be greater for the torso and less for the head. This effectively elevated the head. Combined with a pillow, this may have provided many people with adequate head elevation to avoid some of the ravages of head congestion. However, as mattresses manufacturers began emphasizing bed firmness, the bed became a flatter place to sleep.

Perhaps the flatness of bed design reflects the cultural fact that beds are used for much more than sleeping. Many people read or watch television in bed. Some people eat, work on their lap top computer, or talk on the telephone while in bed. And, of course, people have sex in bed. This requires that the bed be a versatile piece of furniture, and being flat allows for the greatest variety of bed activities. However, this versatility makes the bed less specialized for sleep, which is the primary reason for having a bed. We can eat, work, and play in many other places. We reserve the bed for sleeping. Since that is its primary purpose, it should be best suited for sleeping. And this requires that the head of the bed be elevated.

There are adjustable beds, which can allow a wide variety of bed activities without compromising sleep position. And there are foam wedges for elevating the top portion of the bed. People who have heart failure need gravity to assist lung drainage, as we mentioned. Doctors have prescribed elevating the top part of the body for decades to assist these patients. And doctors have also used wedges and adjustable beds to treat indigestion, where stomach fluid irritates the lower part of the esophagus. Elevating the top of the body allows gravity to assist in keeping stomach juices where they belong.

Yet, when you look at advertisements for beds, the human models in the ads are always sleeping flat and on their sides. Even adjustable beds are shown in advertisements to elevate the head for television watching or reading, but are then shown in the completely flat position for sleeping. This is where our culture is causing us trouble. For some reason, sleep is pictured as something you do flat and on your side.

Snoring and Back Sleeping

A cultural bias towards side sleeping may have to do with snoring. Snoring is considered a particularly unpleasant sound, perhaps because it can disturb a sleeping partner. People ridicule and scoff at the snorer, who sometimes feels so distressed by the criticism that he may seek surgery to remove parts of his mouth and throat to end the nuisance. Some snorers wear an electrical sound detector, usually a gift from a bed partner, which picks up the sound of the offensive snore when it happens, and produces a slight electrical shock. This is supposed to make the snorer change positions and hopefully cease making a racket. It is clear that snoring is a problem for our culture.

When do people snore the loudest? It is when they sleep on their backs. The tongue and soft palate in the mouth can drop back due to gravity and obstruct the airways. This is also the problem with sleep apnea. The flapping of these structures as we try to breathe creates the vibrato of the snore. The cultural stigma against snoring may have been translated into a stigma against back sleeping.

Things would be different if this were a hammock using society. We would all be sleeping on our backs, with our heads above our hearts. But this is a bed society. Bed manufacturers are aware that most people sleep on their sides. That is why they show their ads with side sleepers. They are appealing to the customer, who has certain sleeping preferences. They are selling beds, not trying to reform sleeping behavior. Since most people have poor sleeping posture, many people experience neck and back pain after their 8 hours or so of body compression, congestion, and contortion. Recognizing this, bed manufacturers try to design mattresses that they claim can keep your spine straight. Of course, this must be accomplished with the person sleeping on the side, since this is the culturally preferred position.

Perhaps we can now see the fallacy of this approach. If you want an even spine, then you would want to be on your back. When lying on the side it is very difficult not to curve the spine. The spine consists of interconnected bones, called vertebrae, separated from one another by cartilage discs. Nerves exit the spinal cord through openings between the vertebrae. Curving the spine can cause compression of the discs on one side and impingement of the nerves exiting the vertebrae on that side, as well. We should be able to curve our spine to the left and the right without trouble. But when you sleep on the side you may permanently curve the spine. This compression of the vertebrae can cause back pain and reduced nerve activity, leading to a host of potential problems that your chiropractor will be happy to explain to you.

When you sleep on your back the spine can keep symmetrical and properly adjusted. However, you may experience lower back pain, since the back is not flat but has curves, particularly in the lower back. If you place a pillow underneath your knees, however, this reduces the stress on the lower back. But make sure that the pillow is not cutting off the leg circulation from the knee down.

The Best Sleep Position

In our opinion, the ideal sleeping position is that which you get when in a recliner chair. The head is up, as are the legs. The knees are slightly bent. And you are on your back. Many people fall asleep in their recliners because they are so comfortable. But our culture does not consider recliners sleep furniture. It's not easy putting sheets on them (although we do). And they are usually made for one person, so you'll have to sleep alone (unless you get a loveseat). All this makes people not think about the recliner for sleeping. Too bad, because it really feels wonderful.

Adjustable beds are similar to a large recliner, and can sleep more than one. These would be a good choice for sleeping, apart from their expense. Perhaps as the demand goes up so will the supply, and the price may someday come down.

Insomnia

Of course, throughout this discussion we have been ignoring the length of time a person sleeps. One way to reduce pressure in the head, in addition to head elevation, is to sleep less. Our brains know this. That is why we sometimes awake in the middle of the night with an urge to get up. But the clock says that it's not time to get up. So culture wins over nature, and we stay in bed. Insomnia may simply be a person's brain telling him to get up to relieve the congestion in his head.

The Modern Role of Sleep

If you think that it is difficult to change sleeping behavior, try making someone sleep less. Unless they are extremely motivated, forget it. Sleep for modern man is different than it was for primitive man. We are much more protected from intruders than our primitive ancestors were. We can lock our doors, turn on the porch light, and activate the burglar alarm. We have the luxury of being able to be unconscious for as long as we like. We can even induce unconsciousness with sleeping pills. We don't expect that a hungry grizzly bear will come into our bedroom and eat us while we are dozing. Modern man can sleep longer and deeper than he ever before could. Of course, that means he will suffer more from brain congestion than ever before, too.

For modern people sleep is a rest from our hectic pace of life. We live with phone calls, daily mail, magazines, e-mail, faxes, children, spouses, fellow workers, neighbors, as well as constant stimulation from radios, CD players, television, computers, and movies. The pace of life is getting faster by the day. The only rest we have is in bed. You don't have to drive the kids to soccer practice or dance lessons. You don't have to answer the phone, or cook meals, or go shopping, or deal with business at the office. You can simply slide under the covers, close your eyes, turn off the world, and hopefully have a wonderful dream of a world you wish existed, but doesn't.

For us, sleep is an escape. People want as much of it as they can get. But it shouldn't make them get migraines, or Alzheimer's, or glaucoma, or a stroke. Sleep is meant to be a rest time. It is a time for rejuvenation. It should not be a time for congestion, compression, decay and deterioration.

Your doctor may never have thought of the effect of gravity on brain dysfunction, or the effect of sleep position on the body.

When treating sleep disorders, the doctor is not trained to consider the compression of the body by gravity and its effects on circulation. Why has this obvious fact of the effect of sleep position on human physiology been ignored? Why have so many people suffered unnecessarily, when their salvation may have been as simple as elevating their heads in bed? This brings us to the final chapter, where we can begin to examine the real cause of brain dysfunction and disease.

7

The Real Headache

We have attempted to show the relationship between migraines and various brain and body conditions, all of which may possibly stem from the congestion of the brain due to lying down too flat for too long. It may seem that the number of conditions that can be caused by this congestion, or edema, of the brain makes this an ambitious theory. Actually, we have understated the case.

Too Simplistic?

The brain is responsible for coordinating and initiating virtually all functions of the body. Its nerves and the hormones it secretes stimulate and modulate all of our organs, including the kidneys, gonads, thyroid, lungs, intestines, pancreas, heart, penis, and more. If the brain is congested with fluid and malfunctioning due to low oxygen and sugar levels, all bodily functions will suffer. We could have provided dozens, if not hundreds, of more possible outcomes of brain edema on the body and its health. All of the suggestions we have made are firmly grounded in science and in what is known about the human body. We have refrained from making too many speculations, however, since this may make our theory seem too simplistic. Further, we have not done our own research to prove the point. However, lack of proof does not mean lack of truth.

When it comes to brain dysfunction, the connection to brain edema is clear. The medical literature acknowledges this connection. Even the effect of gravity on the brain has been studied extensively. There has also been research on the differences between standing up and lying down on the physiology of the body. There have been many studies of the effect of tilting the head up or down and to the right or the left on the condition of the brain. (See references) The science is not new. What is new is connecting all these facts and observations to the way we sleep and how this modifies the effect of gravity on our brains.

Considering Culture

Why has this gravity modifying effect of sleeping position been ignored in medical research and treatment? It is because lying flat is considered to be a normal way to sleep. We asked some neurosurgeons and brain physiologists about head elevation and brain edema. They all agreed that head elevation is effective and commonly used to treat brain edema. Why is it not used to *prevent* brain edema? After all, *"If raising the head 30-degrees can reduce brain swelling, then lowering the head to the flat position might create swelling, right"?* The answer they had was that sleeping flat is a normal thing to do. *"Edema cannot be caused by a normal activity"*, they assumed. *"Sleeping flat is something everyone does, so it can't cause disease"*.

Here, then, is the core of the problem. Our cultural behaviors are taken for granted as being normal, and the normal is considered safe. Sleeping flat is a normal practice in our modern culture. It has been falsely assumed that such a common behavior could not create such common problems as migraines, Alzheimer's, sleep apnea, impotence, glaucoma and other products of brain edema.

Actually, sleeping flat is not normal for every culture. Apart from the "primitive sleeper" we presented as a thought experiment, you rarely come across "primitive" societies, where people live with nature, and see the people sleeping flat on the ground for 6-12 hours daily. Insects, snakes, scorpions, and spiders are also on the ground. So are rocks, roots, mud, and morning dew. It also feels hard and uncomfortable lying on the ground or directly on a hard floor. As a result, people who live with nature frequently sleep in hammocks, or on raised "beds" that sag, causing the head to be elevated. Flat sleeping is mostly a product of civilized life — its styles of housing, methods of pest control, and fashions in sleep furniture. And only "civilized" people have the luxury of sleeping for long hours

Because researchers have missed identifying brain edema as an outcome of sleeping position, they have considered head elevation only good for *treating* brain edema, not for *preventing* it. Completing their folly, they have ignored the edema of migraines, Alzheimer's, seizures, and other brain conditions, and have not even recommended head elevation as a treatment. Blinded to this cultural cause of brain edema, they have chosen to ignore the edema altogether.

Unfortunately, this ignorance has cost the public pain, suffering, lives — and money.

Conflict of Interest

It is estimated that 15%-25% of the population suffers from migraines. That translates into about 70 million people in the United States alone. We would call this a huge tragedy. The medical/drug/alternative health industries call it a huge market.

No sane person would ever wish a migraine on someone. But if people are getting migraines, then there will be an industry, or industries, that treats migraines. The demand creates a supply. It's a simple fact of economics.

It's also a simple fact of human nature that if someone profits from the suffering of others, then he is invested in that suffering continuing.

The investment goes beyond the huge sums made selling

migraine treatments. Sleep "experts" should know from the medical literature that sleep apnea is relieved by head elevation. Yet, they usually never mention this simple lifestyle solution, and may recommend surgery of the throat instead. Ophthalmologists should know from the medical literature that glaucoma is related to head elevation. Yet, they prescribe a regimen of lifetime medication instead, requiring continuous office visits for check-ups, and exposing the patient to medication side effects that include heart attacks. And impotence "experts" should know from the medical literature that you can't get the little head up if the big one is too congested. But they are too busy filling prescriptions for Viagra.

Medical Conservatism

History teaches us that medicine is a conservative business that resists new ideas. Changing the minds and treatment patterns of the medical "experts" who make a living treating migraines, Alzheimer's, glaucoma, Parkinson's, sleep disorders, seizures, sex disorders, and other products of a swollen brain will be difficult and may take decades, if it happens at all.

But it can happen.

First, they will have to realize that flat sleeping is not healthy. Many of them personally sleep flat, so they may resist the information since it goes against their personal biases. Unfortunately, people, including doctors, resist change.

Then, they will have to acknowledge that all these various conditions may be different outcomes of the same lifestyle problem. This may be hard for them to do, since they rarely admit that lifestyle has anything to do with health and disease. And the various medical specialties that define their niche by examining the differences between these diseases will not necessarily appreciate the similarities, or the common cause. Even self-evident truths can be ignored.

Of course, the "experts" will also have to rationalize why they have ignored this obvious cause of brain disease, particularly since they have known about this effect of gravity on the brain. Those in authority typically avoid admitting that they are wrong. The first responsibility of authority is to maintain its status. Truth is often a secondary concern.

Finally, they will have to place the health interests of their patients above their personal interests in deriving a living from disease treatment. This issue addresses the character of the practitioner, and some will be better able to leap this hurdle than others.

The "experts" may some day come around to the truth in this report, but don't hold your breath until they do! History teaches us that it can take 20-30 years, if it happens at all. Fortunately, truths are eternal, so they will still be here when people become ready for them.

Actually, the truth of our report should be so self evident that we expect many open-minded doctors will immediately applaud our work and begin recommending that their patients sleep with their heads elevated. The advice is at the worst benign, and at the best curative and preventative of multiple diseases. While some specialists invested in treating a particular disease may act defensively, which is a natural "territorial defense" mechanism, physicians invested more in overall patient care should have no resistance to the simple, obvious fact that people need to sleep with their heads elevated to prevent brain edema.

Specialists

So far we have discussed several possible reasons why this relationship between gravity, sleep behavior, and brain edema has been overlooked by medicine. One reason is the false cultural assumption that flat sleeping is normal and, therefore, cannot cause a health problem. Another reason is that medicine is corrupted by a conflict of interest that favors continuous treatment over prevention and a cure. Additionally, medical conservatism automatically ensures that new ideas will take time to be accepted, despite the toll of suffering caused by the delay. There is one more cause we will now discuss. It relates to medical specialization.

We already mentioned the "divide and conquer" mentality of modern medicine. The whole human body is studied in parts, with little regard for the connections. Specialists study these parts. Each specialty develops its own special medical sub-jargon to discuss its part of the body and to identify its field as a specialty. The more specialties there are, the more the human body becomes divided into parts, creating more confusing jargon and ultimately dividing the entire field of medicine into a Babel of disconnected specialties.

Without focusing on the connections between parts, one specialty may actually have a solution for another specialty's problems, but not know it. This has been the case with brain research. There are many specialties within the category of brain research and disease. Some study migraines. Some study Alzheimer's disease. Some study sleep apnea. Unfortunately, none of these specialists consulted the space medicine specialists who study the effect of zero gravity on the brain. If they had, they would have already realized that flat sleeping is hazardous.

Space medicine is focused on examining the health problems associated with spending time in space, where there is no gravity. What does this do to the body? How can special spacesuits or other devices mitigate this negative effect of zero gravity on the body? These are some of the questions space scientists ask. As a result, they have learned that fluid shifts to the head in space due to zero gravity, causing brain edema, migraines, and other problems. They sometimes simulate this effect on Earth by having people lie flat. In other words, they know that lying flat causes brain edema.

If they were researching brain disease on Earth, then they would have had the answer. But this specialty is focused on space. The researchers who focus on brain disease on Earth don't necessarily read the space medicine literature, so they may never have heard of this zero gravity effect on the brain.

This is the unfortunate outcome of dividing the whole into parts. We have a Humpty-Dumpty medical system, and nobody can put the pieces together again.

The Real Expert

If the specialists can't help, then where can the lay citizen go for answers? Keep this in mind. The wisdom of the forces of nature has culminated in the creation of – you!

Your body was constructed to work well, so long as you don't abuse it. Learn to listen to your bodysense. Listen to its pleasures and pains. These are your guideposts. Learn to hear the voice of health within you. If you feel ill, ask what you have done to cause the illness. How did you get in the way of the operation of your body? What did you do wrong? You must first discover the cause before you can get rid of the problem. And the cause is usually in your behaviors and attitudes. This means it is in your way of life, as taught to you by your culture.

When we were conducting the Migraine Relief Project, we came upon a couple of people with a similar story. After we had told them about our theory regarding head elevation and migraines, they remarked that they had once used a foam wedge under doctor's orders for a different condition, such as indigestion, and, now that they thought about it, they can remember that they didn't have any migraines while on the wedge. Once they returned to normal, flat sleeping, their migraines returned. Their brains told them that head elevation worked. They simply were expecting the answer to come from their doctors, not from themselves.

We expect that many readers will try elevating their heads while sleeping to see the effect. If it works, then they will spread the word to their uncles with memory problems, and their nieces with migraines, and their cousins with glaucoma. In twenty years we may discover that those who had raised their beds in response to this book are spared the devastation of Alzheimer's disease, stroke, Parkinson's disease, and other brain problems.

That would be wonderful, wouldn't it?

The Sleep SELF STUDY

SELF STUDIES are your chance to test for yourself, on yourself, the benefit of a certain lifestyle change. No amount of research on others will ever tell you how this lifestyle change will apply to *you* until *you* try it for yourself. Since the Migraine Relief Project was so successful, we feel that everyone with headaches should try elevating his or her head while sleeping. In addition, this lifestyle solution may also cure glaucoma, sleep apnea, impotence, and seizures, and may help prevent Alzheimer's, stroke, and Parkinson's.

The Sleep SELF STUDY is an ongoing international research project conducted by the SELF STUDY CENTER of the *Institute for the Study of Culturogenic Disease*. Soma and I founded the Institute to further develop the field of applied medical anthropology, and to educate the public on the lifestyle causes of disease and what can be done to live more healthfully. The Institute is a program of the Good Shepherd Foundation, a non-profit research and education organization.

Participation in the Sleep SELF STUDY is cost-free, risk-free, confidential, and open to everyone worldwide. Participants are to raise their beds for 3 months. By that time they will know if it is helping. Those wishing to continue sleeping elevated can enter into the 10-year Alzheimer's Prevention Project, allowing the Institute to track their health over the years to see whether or not their incidence of Alzheimer's is lower than the general, flat public.

How to Elevate Your Head While in Bed

The degree of incline you want is around 30-degrees up from the horizontal, which is about the angle of incline you would have leaning back in a recliner chair. This is the optimum height for your head while sleeping. You will feel more comfortable when lying down, will be able to breathe easier, and will feel less pressure in your head, which is the best way to know that you are helping yourself to better health.

You can elevate your head in bed by using foam wedges for a flat bed, by sleeping on an adjustable bed, or by sleeping on a recliner chair. There are many styles of foam wedges to use. Some wedges are one piece, like a large slice of cheese. You can place the wedge on top of your mattress and cover it with a sheet. Or you can place the wedge underneath the mattress, on top of the box spring. You have a choice of wedge thickness, and we suggest you get the 12-inch thickness, which best achieves a 30-degree elevation. The problem with these wedges, however, is that they tend to make you slide down the incline plane. Placing a pillow underneath your knees can keep you from sliding. The knee pillow also reduces strain on the lower back. Alternatively, there are other types of wedges that come in separate pieces that you position underneath your body to achieve the correct elevation. These may work better for you if the single piece wedge is not working well. Also, some wedges are made from high quality foam, while others use air and are portable. Search the Internet for wedges and you will get an idea of all the choices and prices. They are also available at medical supply stores and foam or mattress shops.

You may need to go to specialty bed stores for adjustable beds. These are mechanically operated, and are the same type of beds that hospitals use. They come in a choice of widths, and would be ideal for head and leg elevation. Their major drawback is their expense. But in the long run, it is cheaper than buying medication to treat migraines.

Many American homes have recliners. These chairs are designed for comfort, and many people fall asleep in them. They come in different sizes, both single and loveseat size, and they recline to different degrees, allowing you to choose the position that feels the most comfortable. Be aware, however, that recliners usually change their position when you move your body. They are stable when they are all the way back, however, so make sure that you are comfortable at that farthest back angle, which is the angle you will be elevated while sleeping. Since each recliner style will have a different farthest back angle, select a new recliner carefully. Get one with the farthest back angle closest to 30-degrees. If you already have a recliner and it does not go back far enough, a pillow underneath your buttocks may help create a better angle. Also, the more padded the recliner, the more comfortable it is to sleep on.

Some people may simply try raising their heads with an extra pillow or two. This may work for some people, but it may close down the windpipe reducing breathing, and may bend the neck too greatly causing muscle pain, misaligned vertebrae, and general discomfort. If you want to try using extra pillows, try to prop up your entire chest, in addition to your head. Keep in mind the body position you would have in a recliner, which is ideal. If you can match this with pillows, then fine.

Also, do not raise the entire bed by putting blocks under the top legs to make the bed higher at the top. This makes the bed a complete incline plane, which will cause blood to pool in your legs and feet. You only want the bed elevated from the middle upwards. Actually, your legs should be slightly elevated, too, as they would be on a recliner. Your legs have been down all day. They need to be up at night to drain.

Whatever your method to elevate your head, *determine to sleep elevated for at least 3 months.* Here are some other tips:

- You can still use a pillow for comfort under your head, but make sure that it does not push against the veins leading from the brain down the sides of the neck. This will congest the brain. Studies have shown that sleeping with the head turned to the right or left reduces brain drainage and increases brain pressure and edema. Therefore, sleep on your back without turning your head to the side.

• Back sleeping will also prevent compression of the breasts, testicles, and penis, which is what happens when you sleep on your side or stomach, as we discussed. This may help women reduce breast tenderness and congestion, as well as help men improve the health and performance of their genitals. So, **the best position is on your back, elevated, with your head facing straight**.

• Avoid pillows that cradle around the neck. They may stabilize the neck vertebrae, but they can also interfere with brain circulation. As we said, you may want to put a pillow underneath your knees to reduce any possible strain on your lower back. You can also help prevent your body from slipping to the side by cradling yourself with pillows. However, make sure that your arms are not leaning on the pillows in such a way that it interferes with circulation.

• If you can get past the cultural bias against sleeping all night on a recliner, then this may work best for you. It does for us. Using a recliner makes a pillow unnecessary, and keeps you from sliding down the incline plane.

• You may want to try extra pillows or an inexpensive wedge first, and then improve your set-up once you are convinced that it is helping you. If you wish, try stuffing a sleeping bag or some rolled up blankets or towels between the mattress and box spring. This substitutes for a wedge. You want the top of the mattress to be raised about 10-12 inches from the box spring, and to taper down from there to be level with the box spring at the waist.

• Of course, you can always sleep in a hammock, which has the added advantage of rocking you to sleep.

Keeping Track of Horizontal Time

• Remember, too, that time spent reclining in a chair to watch television or to read a book is semi-horizontal time that will increase head pressure compared to vertically standing. Therefore, if you sleep 8 hours each night, but before you go to sleep you watch 4 hours of television in a reclining position, then your head has had 8+4=12 hours of horizontal or near horizontal time. Try to keep track of this time you spend awake but not vertical. It will add to your overall head congestion.

• You may also find that you don't need as much sleep after reclining for several hours, since the purpose of sleep is, at least in part, to re-pressurize the head. Reclining may already have partially done that, making it healthier for you to have less sleep.

• The time you spend sitting each day also raises the head pressure relative to standing. If you sit at work all day, and then recline in the evening to read or watch television, your head has not really fully benefited from your vertical time. If you then lie down to sleep, the pressurizing continues. Keep in mind all the time you spend in these head pressurizing positions.

Napping

• This raises the subject of naps. Since the head gets pressurized while sleeping, it follows that 8 hours of continuous pressure may be worse for the head than two separate sessions of 4 hours each. Vertical time in between sleep periods may help alleviate head congestion. So try to sleep less at night and nap during the day, keeping your total hours of sleep the same. People who take naps along with a full night of sleep often wake up with a migraine.

• If your schedule prevents you from taking naps, you may want to simply get up for a while in the middle of the night and then go back to sleep. Breaking up the long night of horizontal time may reduce head congestion and make it easier to sleep.

• Insomnia, like migraines, may be the brain's way of preventing excessive head pressure. Your brain is telling you to get up, since it is getting too congested lying down. Elevating your head may allow you to sleep since it reduces brain congestion.

Massage

• In addition, most people have tight neck muscles. As we explained, this could lead to reduced head circulation, further compromising the brain's oxygen and sugar supplies, and compounding brain edema. To deal with tight neck muscles, try getting a massage. Relaxation techniques may help, but we believe that there is nothing like a massage to relieve muscle pain and tightness. You will need more than one massage. In fact, you will probably need to get into the habit of receiving neck massages, since muscle tightness is a learned phenomenon. Year upon year of stress trains us to tighten our bodies in certain ways. It takes years to overcome these built-in tensions. Learning how to give yourself a massage may help if you do not have someone available to give you one. Self-massage is free, safe, effective, and self-empowering. After you have gone to a massage therapist for a few massages, try to imitate the technique of hand movements on your own neck. You'll be amazed at how easy self-massage is.

• In addition to neck tightness, most people have face and scalp muscle tightness. The muscles of the head are small and numerous, and many of them can become tight as a result of a particular facial expression, compression from sleeping, or injury. Pain in these muscles can feel like a headache, and their tightness may interfere with circulation as it impinges on blood vessels and nerves that pass nearby. Gently massaging your scalp and face can relieve the muscular tension.

Manual Lymph Drainage

•   One form of massage is called manual lymph drainage. This is a specialized massage technique that has been shown to reduce edema in tissues. It is interesting to note that some migraines have been successfully treated by manual lymph drainage. This not only emphasizes the value of massage. It illustrates the fact that edema is causing the migraines.

Chiropractic Adjustments

•   Neck adjustments may also be of value. Tight neck muscles can be the result of vertebrae in the neck being out of adjustment. Tight muscles can also cause the neck to go out of adjustment. It is useful, then, to get a neck adjustment in association with a neck massage. You can learn how to do this by yourself, as well. Soma and I have learned these self-care methods, and it has rewarded us handsomely in reduced neck pain and head congestion.

Exercise

•   Exercise helps to flush and oxygenate the entire body. Some forms of exercise can assist brain drainage, such as bouncing on a rebounder or trampoline. As you descend while bouncing the effect of gravity is reduced, allowing the arterial blood to more easily enter the brain. When you ascend the gravity force is increased, assisting the venous drainage of blood from the brain. Other exercises that capitalize on this "gravity massage" are dancing, skipping, jogging, and swinging on a playground swing. Make sure, however, that you are capable of engaging in these activities. If your spine or neck are out of adjustment, bouncing can irritate the spine, possibly creating tighter muscles and a backache. As with all exercise, you need to be cautious and exercise common sense in what you do. In addition, bending over to pick up things or other bending activities, such as gardening, can also contribute to head pressure. If you want to minimize head congestion, then try to limit these activities.

• In addition, deep breathing flushes your body of carbon dioxide and replenishes oxygen supplies. The negative pressure created in the chest as a result of deep breathing also acts as a pump, pulling blood down from the brain. Whenever you feel brain fatigue or a migraine coming on, try deep breathing to flush and re-oxygenate the brain. Also, drink fruit juices or another good source of sugar to provide energy for your brain.

Tight Clothing

• Finally, avoid tight clothing. Studies have shown that neckties can cause headaches and other problems due to constriction. Clothing should never be tight on any part of the body. This is particularly true for anything worn around the neck. Neckties may be responsible for head congestion. We have not discussed cluster headaches as a separate entity from migraines, since both may merely be different manifestations of the same problem. However, in connection with clothing, it is interesting to note that cluster headaches are more common in men than in women. And men wear neckties more than women do. To wear a necktie, you must button the top shirt collar button. Some shirts have tighter collars than others do. Men who may already have congested brains due to sleeping patterns will be further damaged by a tight collar and necktie. The neck should never be constricted.

• Also, avoid sleeping with tight clothing. Anything with elastic is designed to hold on by constriction and should be avoided. Circulation is more sluggish when we are sleeping, making constrictive clothing even more damaging at that time. Even if there is no elastic, be aware of clothing digging into your body and causing creases, dents, and other marks. Lying on bunched up pajamas or some other material can inhibit circulation, as well. And clothing can interfere with body movement in bed. Try using a warm blanket and skip the pajamas. You may feel wildly free and strange for a little time. But once you get used to the natural freedom, you may never want to sleep textiled again.

The Risks

Are there any risks to sleeping with your head elevated? Studies have shown that head elevation from 25-30 degrees is optimal for brain circulation, and better than lying flat. It has also been shown to reduce brain edema without adversely affecting the brain, heart, or any bodily functions.

Naturally, there are times when any individual needs more or less pressure in the brain. It depends on one's general health status, brain condition, lifestyle activities, degree of dehydration or over-hydration, and the time of day. Lying flat for half an hour may provide necessary re-pressurization of the brain. Some people even do head stands to restore brain pressure. But you would not be wise to stand on your head for 8 hours straight, or to lie flat for that long, either. For general sleeping, an elevation of about 30-degrees offers the best combination of pressure to the head and drainage from the head.

We know of no medical condition that would keep you from trying this experiment of elevating your head slightly while sleeping. But if you have any questions of the appropriateness of you doing this, then we suggest that you consult a health care provider. (You may have to give them this book to read, since this information may be new to them.)

Adjusting to the Change

Some people feel that they cannot sleep elevated, and insist that they are most comfortable when lying flat. Almost all of us have experienced trying to sleep in an aircraft, where the seats only recline to an uncomfortable 70-degrees. If you were uncomfortable trying to sleep on the aircraft, keep in mind that you were not at the optimal angle for reclining. Instead of comparing the comfort of sleeping flat to the discomfort of trying to sleep in an aircraft seat, compare it to sleeping in a recliner chair. (By the way, we have no connection to any recliner companies. We just like how they feel for sleeping, and many people already have them, making recliners ideal for the Sleep SELF STUDY.)

Realize that sleeping positions are learned from childhood. They are notoriously difficult to change. If your mother placed you on your stomach to sleep and turned your head to the right side, then you may feel most comfortable keeping that position all of your life. These early behaviors become etched in our subconscious minds, and altering them raises resistance.

For those who are currently suffering from migraines, there may be less resistance in trying this lifestyle change, since they hope to relieve their suffering. However, when it comes to *preventing* diseases such as Alzheimer's and glaucoma, some people may be more invested in their current flat sleeping behavior than in trying this SELF STUDY. It is always more difficult to get people to prevent a problem than it is to have them treat the problem once it occurs. An ounce of prevention may be worth a pound of cure. But this must be measured against the logic that says, "If it isn't broken, don't fix it."

Perhaps this resistance to head elevation would be less if people realized that sleeping flat is not a natural behavior, as we discussed. People think of flat sleeping as normal, since our culture teaches us to sleep that way. That is the nature of culturogenic diseases. We grow up believing that what we are doing, what our culture has taught us to do, is normal and, therefore, is safe. Statistically it is the norm, since most people in that culture are also doing the same thing. However, what is normal is not necessarily what is healthful.

Finally, expect miracles. We have seen them happen. Some people never have another migraine after raising their heads in bed. But if you have been chronically congesting your brain for decades, it may take time for your brain and body to completely heal. Yet, you will heal. So long as you are alive your body wants to heal, and it can. At the least, elevating the head should immediately slow down, if not reverse, the damaging effects of brain edema, even in cases of Alzheimer's disease and Parkinson's disease. There may be difficulty altering your habitual sleeping patterns, such as wanting to turn over and sleep flat on your stomach. But you will get past these behavioral patterns within a few weeks and will relearn new ones for your new sleeping position.

Of course, nothing works for everyone. But the advice we have just given can do no harm. And it may eliminate migraines, while preventing Alzheimer's disease, Parkinson's disease, and a host of other problems that you don't want.

Contact Us

We would appreciate your notifying us of the results of your SELF STUDY. The Institute is compiling these results to demonstrate the value of this lifestyle solution in the prevention and cure of brain disease. While medical "experts" dislike anecdotal evidence, we love it. It serves the critical purpose of encouraging other people to try the SELF STUDY. The purpose of the SELF STUDY is not only to generate research data. It is to solve the problems of migraines, Alzheimer's, and other brain edema conditions by simply altering lifestyles. We would like to document that this has worked for you.

You can contact us at our mailing address:

The Institute
P.O. Box 1880
Pahoa, Hawaii, USA 96778

Or email us at:

iscd@selfstudycenter.org

You may also benefit from other SELF STUDIES at our SELF STUDY CENTER, which is on the Internet:

www.selfstudycenter.org

We suggest that you become a member of the Institute and receive additional information about new lifestyle solutions to health problems. Contact us for membership information at our email address, or write us.

We hope that this information helps you. You now know the cause of diseases that have confounded researchers for centuries. The solution is simple, perhaps too simple for today's complex world. But truth is usually that way.

Your health, or disease, is now up to you.

Actually, it always has been.

References

The contribution we have made to the understanding of migraines, Alzheimer's disease, and the host of other diseases described in this report is in piecing together information from various medical specialties, and adding to that picture the missing piece of sleep behavior. What follows is a sampling of those separate pieces of the puzzle. We have omitted the names of the authors of these studies for ease of presentation. Readers interested in those names can easily find them through the article title and location we have provided.

We have divided the references into several categories, although there is some overlap. We also provide a glossary of terms for your convenience. It is amazing how medical jargon can complicate and confuse a topic.

First, we will show that head position has been studied extensively in its relation to zero gravity and space research.

SUPINE POSITION and ZERO GRAVITY, MIGRAINES, BRAIN EDEMA

Because of a lack of gravity in space, fluid shifts to the head and causes brain edema and migraines. As we already discussed, scientists studying this effect simulate it here on Earth by having people lie flat with their heads turned various ways. They know that a head lying flat gets brain edema. But they never applied that knowledge to the prevention or treatment of brain edema conditions, or to sleep behavior. This research is done by brain physiologist specialists who do not necessarily apply their findings to the problems of other medical specialties, such as those studying headaches.

Glossary:

Antiorthostatic hypokinesia = lying down without moving (bedrest)
Hemodynamics = what's happening to the blood supply
Microgravity = no gravity, as in outer space
Supine = flat on the back

Effect of head-down tilt on brain water distribution.
Eur J Appl Physiol. 1999 Mar;79(4):367-73.

[Some physiological effects caused by 30 days of bed rest in different body positions].
Kosm Biol Aviakosm Med. 1980 Jul-Aug;14(4):55-8.

[Various reactions of the human body during 7 days of anti-orthostatic hypokinesia].
Kosm Biol Aviakosm Med. 1986 Jan-Feb;20(1):29-32.

Effect of antiorthostatic bed rest on hepatic blood flow in man.
Aviat Space Environ Med. 1988 Apr;59(4):306-8.

[Clinical aspects of a change in the nervous system after 49-day head-down hypokinesis].
Kosm Biol Aviakosm Med. 1977 Nov-Dec;11(6):26-31.

[30-day experiment in modelling the physiological effects of weightlessness].
Kosm Biol Med. 1972 Jul-Aug;6(4):26-8.

Redistribution of blood flow in the cerebral cortex of normal subjects during head-up postural change.
Clin Auton Res. 1992 Apr;2(2):119-24.

Body volume changes during simulated microgravity. II: Comparison of horizontal and head-down bed rest.
Aviat Space Environ Med. 1993 Oct;64(10):899-904.

Effect of a central redistribution of fluid volume on response to lower-body negative pressure.
Aviat Space Environ Med. 1990 Jan;61(1):38-42.

Simulated microgravity increases cutaneous blood flow in the head
and leg of humans.
Aviat Space Environ Med. 1995 Sep;66(9):872-5.

Recent bed rest results and countermeasure development at NASA.
Acta Physiol Scand Suppl. 1994;616:103-14. Review.

Transcapillary fluid shifts in tissues of the head and neck during and
after simulated microgravity.
J Appl Physiol. 1991 Dec;71(6):2469-75.

Effect of simulated weightlessness on the postural response of
microvascular cutaneous blood flow.
Physiologist. 1990 Feb;33(1 Suppl):S54-5.

 Postural variations of intraocular pressure—preflight experiments for
the D1-mission.
Ophthalmic Res. 1986;18(1):55-60.

[Antiorthostatic hypokinesia as an approximate model of
weightlessness].
Kosm Biol Aviakosm Med. 1979 Jan-Feb;13(1):23-8.

[Clinico-physiological aspects of the tissue oxygen supply of the
human body during head-down tilt hypokinesia].
Kosm Biol Aviakosm Med. 1988 Mar-Apr;22(2):45-9.

Altered autonomic regulation of cardiac function during head-up tilt
after 28-day head-down bed-rest with counter-measures.
Clin Physiol. 1994 May;14(3):291-304.

Antiorthostatic hypokinesia as a method of weightlessness simulation.
Aviat Space Environ Med. 1976 Oct;47(10):1083-6.

[30-day experiment in modelling the physiological effects of
weightlessness. Organization of the experiments and general condition
of the test subjects].
Kosm Biol Med. 1972 Jul-Aug;6(4):28-32.

Response of the circadian system to 6 degrees head-down tilt bed rest.
Aviat Space Environ Med. 1993 Jan;64(1):50-4.

Twenty-four hours of bed rest with head-down tilt: venous and arteriolar changes of limbs.
Am J Physiol. 1991 Apr;260(4 Pt 2):H1043-50.

[Central and general hemodynamics in healthy persons during simulated weightlessness].
Kosm Biol Aviakosm Med. 1990 Jan-Feb;24(1):15-7. Russian.

Intraocular pressure and retinal vascular changes during transient exposure to microgravity.
Am J Ophthalmol. 1993 Mar 15;115(3):347-50.

Heart volume during short-term head-down tilt (-6 degrees) in comparison with horizontal body position.
Aviat Space Environ Med. 1987 Sep;58(9 Pt 2):A61-3.

[Body fluids during 120-day anti-orthostatic hypokinesia].
Kosm Biol Aviakosm Med. 1989 Sep-Oct;23(5):57-61.

The vascular basis of the positional influence of the intraocular pressure.
Albrecht Von Graefes Arch Klin Exp Ophthalmol. 1978 May 2;206(2):99-106.

Postural behaviour of intraocular pressure in diabetics.
Br J Ophthalmol. 1986 Jun;70(6):456-9.

Postural responses of head and foot cutaneous microvascular flow and their sensitivity to bed rest.
Aviat Space Environ Med. 1991 Mar;62(3):246-51.

Cerebral blood velocity and other cardiovascular responses to 2 days of head-down tilt.
J Appl Physiol. 1993 Jan;74(1):319-25.

Pulmonary tissue volume, cardiac output, and diffusing capacity in sustained microgravity.
J Appl Physiol 1997 Sep;83(3):810-6

Fluid Shifts in vascular and extravascular spaces during and after simulated weightlessness.
Med Sci Sports Exerc 1983;15(5):421-7

Characteristics of the sleep of men in simulated space flights.
Avait Space Environ Med 1975 Apr;46(4 Sec 1):401-8

Effects of head-down tilt and saline loading on body weight, fluid, and electrolyte homeostasis in man.
Acta Physiol Scand Suppl 1992;604:13-22

Body volume changes during simulated microgravity I:Technique and comparison of men and women during horizontal bed rest.
Avait Space Environ Med 1993 Oct;64(10):893-8

[Specific aspects of the nervous system and the brain blood supply in women during prolonged anti-orthostatic hypokinesia]. Russian
Aviakosm Ekolog Med 1999;33(2):9-12

Effect of head down tilt on brain water distribution.
Eur J Appl Physiol 1999 Mar;79(4):367-73

Effect of simulated weightlessness on the response characteristics of human brain.
Sci China [B] 1989 Nov;32(11):1329-41

Simulation of space flight with whole-body head-down tilt: influence on intraocular pressure and retinocortical processing.
Avait Space Environ Med 1987 Sep;58(9 Pt 2):A139-42

[Hemodynamic and cerebral ventricular functions during head-down tilt at –15 degrees]. Russian
Kosm Biol Aviakosm Med 1985 Mar-Apr;19(2):39-42

[Prognostic importance of the head-down tilting load]. Russian
Koam Biol Aviakosm Med 1980 May-Jun;14(3):48-54

MIGRAINES and BRAIN EDEMA, BRAIN CIRCULATION, AND RELATED CONDITIONS

Now we will show that researchers know that migraines are associated with brain circulation problems, brain edema, low brain oxygen, low brain sugar, and with other brain edema conditions.

Glossary:

ataxia = lack of muscular coordination
cephalic = brain
cerebrospinal fluid pleocytosis = increased white blood cells (lymphocytes) in spinal fluid
CSF = cerebrospinal fluid
etiology = cause
hemicrania = pain on one side of the head
hemiplegia = paralysis on one side of the body
hydrocephalus = water on the brain
hyperemia = excess blood; congestion
hypoglycemia = low glucose (sugar)
hypoxia = low oxygen
intracranial = inside the brain
ischemia = lack of blood in an area of the body due to mechanical obstruction or functional constriction of a blood vessel
paroxysmal = sudden onset
pathogenesis = origin and development of disease
reactive hyperemia = excessive return of blood
stenosis = abnormal constriction of a channel or opening
thrombopenia = low platelet count
vasodilation = opening up of a blood vessel

Ischemia may be the cause of neurological deficits in classic migraine.
Arch Neurol. 1990 Feb;47(2):124-7.

Is there a need for alternative approaches in the therapy of cerebrovascular disorders?
Eur Neurol. 1986;25 Suppl 1:7-26.

Discussion, ideas abound in migraine research; consensus remains elusive.
JAMA. 1987 Jan 2;257(1):9-12.

Migraine and intracranial swelling.
Lancet. 1985 Dec 7;2(8467):1308-9.

Migraine, a result of increased CSF pressure: a new pathophysiological concept.
Proceedings of Second International Headache Congress (June 18-21, 1985):96-97

Migraine and intracranial swelling: an experiment of nature.
Lancet. 1985 Sep 28;2(8457):718.

The regulation of cerebral blood flow - its relationship to migraine.
Arch Neurobiol (Madr). 1974;37 SUPPL:15-25.

[Cortical edema in hemoplegic migraine].
Ugeskr Laeger. 1984 Jun 18;146(25):1861-3.

[Cerebral ischemic accidents during migraine attacks. A report on "complicated migraine"].
Rev Neurol (Paris). 1980;135(12):867-84.

Migraine associated with focal cerebral edema, cerebrospinal fluid pleocytosis, and progressive cerebellar ataxia: MRI documentation.
Neurology. 1990 Aug 1;40(8):1284

Letter: Hemiplegic migraine: cerebrospinal fluid abnormalities.
J Pediatr. 1974 Jul;85(1):139.

The ischemic hypotheses of migraine.
Arch Neurol. 1987 Mar;44(3):321-2.

Migraine: theories of pathogenesis.
Lancet. 1992 May 16;339(8803):1202-7.

Menstrual migraine.
Headache. 1992 Jun;32(6):312-3.

Migraine and intracranial vascular malformations.
Headache. 1994 May;34(5):287.

Migraine: a cerebral disorder.
Lancet. 1984 Jul 14;2(8394):86-9.

[Migraine and regional cerebral blood flow].
Nord Med. 1985;100(11):284-5.

Effect of chocolate on migraine: a double-blind study.
J Neurol Neurosurg Psychiatry 1974;37:445-48

Effort, high altitude and decompression headache. In: Cerebral hypoxia
in the pathogenesis of migraine. London: Pitman, 1982:28-35

Migraine headache and survival in women.
Br Med J 1988;287:1442-43

Headaches in insulin dependent diabetic patients.
Headache 1989;29:660-63

On megrim, sick-headache and some allied disorders: a contribution to
the pathology of nerve storms.
London: Churchill, 1873:26

Cephalic hyperemia during migraine headaches. A prospective study.
Headache. 1986 Sep;26(8):388-97.

Vasodilatation and migraine.
Lancet. 1990 Apr 7;335(8693):822-3. Review.

Chronic vasoconstriction may have role in migraine headaches.
Arch Intern Med. 1980 Jan;140(1):19.

Reactive hyperaemia and migraine.
Lancet. 1981 Aug 8;2(8241):305.

[Migraine and trauma].
Wien Z Nervenheilkd Grenzgeb. 1969;27(1):45-76.

Diabetes and migraine.
Lancet. 1970 Aug 15;2(7668):369.

Cerebral artery spasm and migraine.
Lancet. 1990 Feb 24;335(8687):480-1.

Migraines and the sinuses, report on 441 cases.
Rhinol Suppl. 1992;14:111-5.

Paroxysmal hypertensive hemicrania.
Headache. 1977 Mar;17(1):5-6.

Valproate-withdrawal induced migraine.
Headache. 1994 Jul-Aug;34(7):445.

Migraine as a defect of brain oxidative metabolism: a hypothesis.
J Neurol. 1989 Feb;236(2):124-5.

The reversible posterior cerebral edema syndrome.
AJNR Am J Neuroradiol. 1998 Mar;19(3):591.

Migraine and premenstral syndrome.
Cephalalgia. 1993 Dec;13(6):377.

Focal neurological deficits and migraine at high altitude.
J Neurol Neurosurg Psychiatry. 1995 May;58(5):637.

Prevalence of migraine in patients with diabetes.
Br Med J (Clin Res Ed). 1985 Feb 9;290(6466):467-8.

Regional cerebral blood flow and oxygen metabolism during migraine
with and without aura.
Cephalalgia. 1997 Aug;17(5):570-9.

Vestibular disorders in patients with migraine.
Eur Arch Otorhinolaryngol Suppl. 1997;1:S55-7.

Basilar artery migraine and reversible imaging abnormalities.
AJNR Am J Neuroradiol. 1998 Jun-Jul;19(6):1116-9.

Case report: transient unilateral cerebral oedema in hemiplegic
migraine: MR imaging and angiography.
Clin Radiol. 1996 Jan;51(1):72-6.

Migraine coma. Meningitic migraine with cerebral oedema associated
with a new form of autosomal dominant cerebellar ataxia.
Brain. 1985 Sep;108 (Pt 3):555-77.

Migraine and somnambulism.
Aust N Z J Med. 1993 Dec;23(6):715

[A severe ophthalmologic complication of migraine]. French
Bull Soc Ophthalmol Fr. 1986 Oct;86(10):1199-200

Migraine and oral contraception.
Drug Ther Bull. 1987 Nov 30;25(24):95-6

[Thrombopenia and migraine. Parallel course of 2 diseases]. French
Presse Med. 1986 Jan 11;15(1):33-4

Acquired learning problems secondary to migraine.
J Dev Behav Pediatr. 1982 Dec;3(4):247-8

Transient global amnesia and migraine.
Neurology. 1983 Aug;33(8):1106-7

Small blood vessels in migraine.
Lancet. 1970 Oct 17;2(7677):832

Whiplash and its relationship to migraine.
Headache. 1987 Sep;27(8):452-7

[Migraine and thrombocytopenia]. German
Dtsch Med Wochenschr. 1988 Mar 4;113(9):363-4

Is a migraine patient more sensitive to stressors? A
neuropsychological and neurophysiological study.
Electromyogr Clin Neurophysiol. 1988 Nov-Dec;28(7-8):405-8

Method of precipitating and preventing some migraine attacks.
Br Med J. 1966 Nov 19;2(524):1242-3

Is there a difference between classic and common migraine? What is
migraine, after all?
Arch Neurol. 1985 Mar;42(3):275-6

Weekend migraine in men.
Lancet. 1992 Jan 4;339(8784):67

Hyperventilation during migraine attacks.
Br Med J. 1980 May 24;280(6226):1254

Migraine: then and now.
Med J Aust. 1996 May 6;164(9):519-20

The link between migraine and dizziness.
Headache. 1993 Mar;33(3):162-3

Cerebral hypoperfusion followed by hyperperfusion in classic migraine.
Arch Neurol. 1989 Jun;46(6):605-6

The cerebral etiology of high-altitude cerebral edema and acute mountain sickness.
Wilderness Environ Med. 1999 Summer;10(2):97-109

Hypoglycemic migraine.
Mo Med. 1975 Apr;72(4):194-7

Migraine: Avoiding trigger factors.
Nurs Mirror. 1977 Aug 11;145(6):18-20

Changes in regional cerebral blood flow during the course of classic migraine attacks.
Ann Neurol. 1983; 13:633-41

Cerebrospinal-fluid abnormalities associated with migraine.
Med J Aust. 1984 Sep 29;141(7):459-61

Vasodilation and migraine.
Lancet. 1990 Apr 7;335(8693):822-3

Cerebral blood flow in migraine.
Headache. 1977 Sep;17(4):148-52

Migraine and weather.
Headache. 1979 Nov;19(7):375-8

Preventing migraine: a study of precipitating factors.
Headache. 1988 Aug;28(7):481-3

Exercise induced migraine.
Ir Med J. 1990 Sep;83(3):126

Migraine with aura and migraine without aura are not different entities.
Cephalalgia. 1995 Jun;15(3):186-90

Unraveling the migraine mystery.
J AM Osteopath Assoc. 1990 Oct;90(10):866

Computerised axial tomography findings in patients with migrainous headaches.
Br Med J. 1976 Jul 17;2(6028)149-50

Migraine due to hydrocephalus.
Headache. 1984 Sep;24(5):272-3

Diet and migraine: a review of the literature.
J Am Diet Assoc. 1983 Oct;83(4):459-63

[Cerebral atherosclerosis and the cervical migraine symptom complex].
Russian
Kiln Med (Mosk). 1967 Sep;45(9):79-82

Prevention of exercise induced migraine by quantitative warm-up.
Headache. 1985 Sep;25(6):317-9

Migraine and cerebral hypoxia: a hypothesis with pharmacotherapeutic implications.
Cephalagia. 1985 May; 5 Suppl 2:131-3

Goggle migraine.
N Engl J Med. 1983 Jan 27;308(4):226-7

Migraine, headache, and survival in women.
Br Med J. (Clin Res Ed). 1983 Dec 3;287(6406):1718

Migraine with aura, cerebral ischemia, spreading depression, and compton scatter.
Headache. 1991 Jan;31(1):49-53

A study of migraine in pregnancy.
Neurology. 1972 Aug;22(8):824-8

Cerebrospinal fluid (CSF) investigations in migraine.
Cephalalgia. 1989 Mar;9(1):53-7

[Is migraine an allergic disease]? French
Presse Med. 1989 Mar 4;18(9):459-61

Dietary causes of migraine.
Chem Ind. 1970 Feb 7;6:173

Migraine, migrainous, migrainoid…
Headache. 1987 Sep;27(8):465-6

The anatomy of migraine.
Eye Ear Nose Throat Mon. 1974 Feb;53(2):69-73

Diabetes and migraine.
Lancet 1970 Aug 15;2(7668):369

Effect of diabetes on migraine.
Lancet. 1970 Aug 1;2(7666):241-3

Prevalence of migraine in patients with diabetes.
Br Med J (Clin Res Ed). 1984 Dec 8;289(6458):1579-80

[Manual lymph drainage in migraine treatment – a pathophysiological
explanatory model]. German
Z Lymphol 1989 Jul;13(1):48-53

[Lymph drainage and edema therapy using physical drainage
treatment]. German
Z Lymphol 1980 Sep;4(2):67-75

Relief of common migraine by exercise [letter].
J Neurol Neurosurg Psychiatry 1987 Dec;50(12):1700-1

An elderly black woman with a painful, "swollen" face.
Ann Allergy 1985 Dec;55(6):771, 819-24

Swelling at the site of a skull defect during migraine headache.
J Neurol Neurosurg Psychiatry. 1995 Dec;59(6):641

Subcutaneous blood flow in the temporal region of migraine patients.
Acta Neurol Scand 1987 May;75(5):310-8

Cardiovascular and biochemical assessment in migraine patients
submitted to tilt test.
Funct Neurol. 1986 Jul-Sep;1(3):285-90

Regional cerebral blood flow during migraine attacks by Xenon-133
inhalation and emission tomography.
Brain. 1984 Jun;107 (Pt 2):447-61

Cerebral blood flow velocities are reduced during attacks of unilateral migraine without aura.
Cephalalgia. 1995 Apr;15(2):109-16

Is ischemia involved in the pathogenesis of migraine?
Pathol Biol (Paris) 1982 May;30(5):318-24

Pathogenesis of migraine: the biobehavioural and hypoxia theories reconciled.
Acta Neurol Belg. 1994;94(2):79-86

Cerebral blood flow asymmetries in headache-free migraineurs.
Stroke 1987 Nov-Dec;18(6):1164-5

Cerebral blood flow in migraine and cortical spreading depression.
Acta Neurol Scand Suppl 1987;113:1-40

Migraine and depression: biological aspects.
J Psychiatr Res 1993 Apr-Jun;27(2):223-31

Effects of body heat and mental arithmetic on facial sweating and blood flow in unilateral migraine headache.
Psychophysiology 1991 Mar;28(2):172-6

Bilateral retinal hemorrhages and disk edema in migraine.
Am J Ophthalmol. 1977 Oct;84(4):555-8

Impairment of cerebral serotonin and energy metabolism during ischemia: relevance to migraine.
Adv Neurol. 1982;33:35-40

Arterial stenosis in migraine: spasm or arteriopathy?
Headache. 1990 Jan;30(2):52-61

Pathophysiology of migraine—new insights.
Can J Neurol Sci. 1999 Nov;26 Suppl 3:S12-9

ALZHEIMER'S and MIGRAINES, BRAIN BLOOD FLOW, BRAIN EDEMA

The following shows that Alzheimer's disease is associated with brain edema, reduced brain circulation, and is linked with migraines.

Glossary:

cerebrovascular = blood supply of the brain
embolic = relating to a plug within a blood vessel
ischemia = lack of blood in an area of the body due to mechanical obstruction or functional constriction of a blood vessel
MRI = magnetic resonance imaging, a type of radiological procedure
orthostatic hypotension = low blood pressure upon rising to the upright position
tomography = a type of X-ray procedure

Intracranial space-occupying lesions in patients attending a migraine clinic.
Practitioner. 1985 May;229(1403):477-81.

Age-related cerebrovascular disease alters the symptomatic course of migraine.
Cephalalgia. 1998 May;18(4):202-8; discussion 171.

Alzheimer's disease risk factors as related to cerebral blood flow.
Med Hypotheses 1996 Apr;46(4):367-77

[Migraine and dementia].
Ugeskr Laeger. 1980 May 19;142(21):1346-7. Danish

Cortical CSF volume fluctuations by MRI in brain aging, dementia and hydrocephalus.
Neuroreport 1994 Sep 8:5(14):1699-704

Orthostatic hypotension in Alzheimer's disease: result or cause of brain dysfunction?
Clin Auton Res 1996 Feb;6(1):29-36

Cerebral microischemia as a potential precipitant of the neurodegenerative cascade of Alzheimer's disease.
Ann N Y Acad. Sci. 1997 Sep 26;826:437-9. Review

[Alzheimer's disease and diabetes: are they bedfellows]?
Rev Med Univ Navarra. 1997 Jan-Mar;41(1):46-57. Review.

Microembolic brain injuries from cardiac surgery: are they seeds of future
Alzheimer's disease?
Ann N Y Acad Sci. 1997 Sep 26;826:386-9. Review.

Functional imaging of blood brain barrier permeability by single photon
emission computerized tomography and positron emission tomography.
Adv Tech Stand Neurosurg. 1992;19:103-19. Review.

The types of headaches that affect the elderly.
Geriatrics. 1976 Sep;31(9):103-6.

Cerebrospinal fluid production is reduced in healthy aging.
Neurology. 1990 Mar;40(3 Pt 1):500-3.

CSF in Alzheimer's disease. Studies on blood-brain barrier function and
intrathecal protein synthesis.
J Neurol Sci. 1985 Aug;70(1):73-80.

Age dependency of resistance to cerebrospinal fluid outflow.
J Neurosurg. 1998 Aug;89(2):275-8.

[Relation between resorption resistance of cerebrospinal fluid and the
degree of intracranial pressure].
Pol Tyg Lek. 1992 Apr 6-13;47(14-15):314-6. Polsh.

Decrease of cerebrospinal fluid flow with increasing age.
Neuroradiology. 1978 Feb 17;14(5):275-7.

Transport and production of cerebrospinal fluid (CSF) change in aging
humans under normal and diseased conditions.
Z Gerontol. 1993 Jul-Aug;26(4):251-5.

Intracranial pressure and conductance to outflow of cerebrospinal fluid in
normal-pressure hydrocephalus.
J Neurosurg. 1979 Apr;50(4):489-93.

MR imaging of the hippocampus in normal pressure hydrocephalus:
correlations with cortical Alzheimer's disease confirmed by pathologic
analysis.
AJNR Am J Neuroradiol. 2000 Feb;21(2):409-14.

Prevalence of Alzheimer's disease in patients investigated for presumed normal pressure hydrocephalus: a clinical and neuropathological study.
Acta Neurochir (Wien). 1999;141(8):849-53.

Pathology of cerebrospinal fluid and interstitial fluid of the CNS: significance for Alzheimer disease, prion disorders and multiple sclerosis.
J Neuropathol Exp Neurol. 1998 Oct;57(10):885-94. Review.

MR differential diagnosis of normal-pressure hydrocephalus and Alzheimer disease: significance of perihippocampal fissures.
AJNR Am J Neuroradiol. 1998 May;19(5):813-9.

Magnetic resonance imaging of the ageing brain.
East Afr Med J. 1997 Oct;74(10):656-9. Review.

[Single photon emission computed tomography in the diagnosis of Alzheimer's disease].
Nippon Ronen Igakkai Zasshi. 1997 Jun;34(6):468-73. Japanese.

Functional brain imaging with single-photon emission computed tomography in the diagnosis of Alzheimer's disease.
Int Psychogeriatr. 1997;9 Suppl 1:223-7; discussion 247-52.

Single SPECT measures of cerebral cortical perfusion reflect time-index estimation of dementia severity in Alzheimer's disease.
J Nucl Med. 2000 Jan;41(1):57-64.

Positron emission tomography for diagnosis of Alzheimer's disease and vascular dementia.
J Neural Transm Suppl. 1998;53:237-50. Review.

The differential diagnosis of Alzheimer's disease. Cerebral atrophy versus normal pressure hydrocephalus.
Neuroimaging Clin N Am. 1995 Feb;5(1):19-31. Review.

Brain inflammation in Alzheimer disease and the therapeutic implications.
Curr Pharm Des. 1999 Oct;5(10):821-36. Review.

Pharmacologic management of Alzheimer disease part III: nonsteroidal antiinflammatory drugs—emerging protective evidence?
Ann Pharmacother. 1999 Jul-Aug;33(7-8):840-9. Review.

[Epidemiology and risk factors of Alzheimer's disease].
Vestn Ross Akad Med Nauk. 1999;(1):39-46. Review. Russian.

The importance of inflammatory mechanisms in Alzheimer disease.
Exp Gerontol. 1998 Aug;33(5):371-8. Review.

Inflammation of the brain in Alzheimer's disease: implications for therapy.
J Leukoc Biol. 1999 Apr;65(4):409-15. Review.

Anti-inflammatory drugs and Alzheimer-type pathology in aging.
Neurology. 2000 Feb 8;54(3):732-4.

Mechanisms of cell death in Alzheimer disease—immunopathology.
J Neural Transm Suppl. 1998;54:159-66. Review.

Importance of immunological & inflammatory processes in the pathogenesis
and therapy of Alzheimer's disease.
Int J Neurosci. 1998 Sep;95(3-4):203-36. Review.

[Inflammatory mechanisms in the pathogenesis of Alzheimer's disease].
Tijdschr Gerontol Geriatr. 1997 Oct;28(5):213-8. Review. Dutch.

The inflammatory response system of brain: implications for therapy of
Alzheimer and other neurodegenerative diseases.
Brain Res Brain Res Rev. 1995 Sep;21(2):195-218. Review.

Inflammatory pathogenesis in Alzheimer's disease: biological mechanisms&
cognitive sequeli.
Neurosci Biobehav Rev. 1999 May;23(5):615-33. Review.

Anti-inflammatory substances - a new therapeutic option in Alzheimer's
disease.
Drug Discov Today. 1999 Jun;4(6):275-282.

The importance of inflammatory mechanisms for the development of
Alzheimer's disease.
Exp Gerontol. 1999 Jun;34(3):453-61. Review.

Inflammation and Alzheimer's disease pathogenesis.
Neurobiol Aging. 1996 Sep-Oct;17(5):681-6. Review.

Inflammation and Alzheimer's disease: mechanisms & therapeutic strategies.
Gerontology. 1997;43(1-2):143-9. Review.

Inflammation and Alzheimer's disease: relationships between pathogenic
mechanisms and clinical expression.
Exp Neurol. 1998 Nov;154(1):89-98. Review.

STROKE and MIGRAINES, ISCHEMIA

We will now show the link between stroke and migraines.

Glossary:

cerebral vascular accident = stroke
focal cerebral ischemia = low blood supply to a small area of the brain
hemicrania = pain on one side of the head
infarction = an area of dead tissue caused by blocked blood vessels leading to the area
neurogenic ischemia = low blood supply in the brain
vertebrobasilar ischemia = low blood supply to the back of the brain

Migrainous stroke.
Stroke. 1988 Oct;19(10):1306.

Migraine as a model of neurogenic ischemia.
Headache. 1982 Nov;22(6):287-8.

Migraine-related stroke in childhood.
Lancet. 1991 Jun 22;337(8756):1546-7.

Ischemic strokes and migraine.
Neuroradiology. 1985;27(6):583-7.

[Migraine, a risk factor for ischemic cerebral stroke].
Med Welt. 1983 Feb 25;34(8):233-4.

Ischemic stroke and migraine in childhood: coincidence or causal relation?
J Child Neurol. 1999 Jul;14(7):451-5. Review.

Vertebrobasilar ischaemia.
QJM. 1998 Dec;91(12):799-811. Review.

History of migraine and risk of cerebral ischaemia in young adults. The Italian National Research Council Study Group on Stroke in the Young. Lancet. 1996 Jun 1;347(9014):1503-6.

Cerebral blood flow in migraine accompaniments and vertebrobasilar ischemia.
Stroke. 1994 Jun;25(6):1219-22.

Severe diffuse intracranial vasospasm as a cause of extensive migrainous cerebral infarction.
Cephalalgia. 1993 Aug;13(4):289-92.

Migrainous stroke.
Cephalalgia. 1993 Aug;13(4):231.

Basilar artery migraine or cerebral vascular accident?
J Manipulative Physiol Ther. 1993 Jun;16(5):354-5.

Ischaemia-induced (symptomatic) migraine attacks may be more frequent than migraine-induced ischaemic insults.
Brain. 1993 Feb;116 (Pt 1):187-202.

[Platelets and migraine].
Pathol Biol (Paris). 1992 Apr;40(4):305-12. Review.

Migraine and vertebrobasilar ischemia.
Neurology. 1991 Jan;41(1):55-61.

Stroke as a complication of migraine disease.
J Indiana State Med Assoc 1981 Aug;74(8):506-8

A controlled study of ischemic stroke risk in migraine patients.
J Clin Epidemiol 1989;42(8):773-80

Migrainous stroke.
Cephalalgia. 1993 Aug;13(4):231

Life-threatening Migraine.
Arch Neurol. 1982 Jun;39(6):374-6

Neurological manifestations of migraine.
Heart Dis Stroke. 1993 Sep-Oct;2(5):422-3

Migrainous cerebral infarction [editorial].
Br Med J. 1977 Feb 26;1(6060):532-3

Focal cerebral ischemia and migraine.
Cephalalgia. 1985 May;5 Suppl 2:21-2

[Cerebrovascular accidents and migraine]. French
Ann Med Interne (Paris). 1983;134(4):306-9
[Hemicrania and cerebral ischemia in young adults]. Italian
Riv Neurol. 1986 Mar-Apr;56(2):106-12

[Cerebral ischemic accidents during migraine attacks. A report on
"complicated migraine"]. French
Rev Neurol (Paris) 1980;135(12):867-84

[Cerebral complications in migraine]. Polish
Przegl Lek. 1966;22(11):708-10

[Multiple cerebral infarctions during a migraine attack]. Spanish
Neurologia. 1991 Feb;6(2):68-70

Cerebral infarction in patients with migraine accompaniments.
Headache. 1988 Oct;28(9):599-601

GLAUCOMA and MIGRAINES, HEAD AND BODY POSITION, AND EYE PRESSURE

The glaucoma researchers deliberately examined the pressure in the eyes as a result of head elevation. There is no charitable explanation why head elevation has not been routinely recommended for glaucoma prevention and treatment.

Glossary:

intraocular = in the eyes
neuropathy = disease of the nervous system

Altering body position affects intraocular pressure and visual function.
Invest Ophthalmol Vis Sci. 1988 Oct;29(10):1492-7.

The influence of posture on intraocular pressure.
Indian J Ophthalmol. 1981 Apr;29(1):1-3.

Increased intraocular pressure with head-down position.
Am J Ophthalmol. 1984 Jul 15;98(1):114-5.

Diurnal variation of intraocular pressure and the overriding effects of sleep.
Am J Optom Physiol Opt. 1987 Jan;64(1):54-61.

Intraocular pressure, ocular pulse pressure, and body position.
Am J Optom Physiol Opt. 1985 Jan;62(1):59-62.

Intraocular pressure, retinal vascular, and visual acuity changes during 48 hours of 10 degrees head-down tilt.
Aviat Space Environ Med. 1990 Sep;61(9):810-3.

Effect of seasons upon intraocular pressure in healthy population of China.
Korean J Ophthalmol. 1996 Jun;10(1):29-33.

Retinal vessel responses to passive tilting.
Eye. 1990;4 (Pt 5):751-6.

Pressure differential of intraocular pressure measured between supine and sitting position.
Ann Ophthalmol. 1981 Mar;13(3):323-6.

Effect of inverted body position on intraocular pressure.
Am J Ophthalmol. 1984 Dec 15;98(6):784-7.

[Experimental studies on the effect of the intraocular pressure on the retinal microcirculation in vivo. 2. Influences of induced intraocular hypertension].
Nippon Ganka Gakkai Zasshi. 1973 Jul;77(7):626-36.

Effect of body position on intraocular pressure and aqueous flow.
Invest Ophthalmol Vis Sci. 1987 Aug;28(8):1346-52.

[Are there genuine and pseudo-normal pressure glaucoma? Body position-dependent intraocular pressure values in normal pressure glaucoma].
Klin Monatsbl Augenheilkd 1997 Oct;211(4):235-40. German.

Migraine and tension headache in high-pressure and normal-pressure glaucoma.
Am J Ophthalmol 2000 Jan;129(1):102-4

Influence of body position on the intraocular pressure of normal and glaucomatous eyes.
Ophthalmologica 1975;171(2):132-45

Influence of posture on the visual field in glaucoma patients and controls.
Ophthalmologica 1995;209(3):129-31

Bilateral sequential migrainous ischemic optic neuropathy.
Am J Ophthalmol. 1985 Apr 15;99(4):489.

Simulation of spaceflight with whole-body head-down tilt: influence on intraocular pressure and retinocortical processing.
Aviat Space Environ Med. 1987 Sep;58(9 Pt 2):A139-42.

SLEEP APNEA and SLEEP POSITION

The sleep apnea field has also directly studied head elevation. Several studies have discovered that sleep apnea is cured by head elevation. Yet, this knowledge is hardly ever mentioned. When does medical negligence become medical conspiracy?

Glossary:

idiopathic = denoting a disease of unknown cause
papilledema = swelling of the optic nerve due to increased intracranial pressure

Therapeutic effect of posture in sleep apnea.
South Med J. 1986 Sep;79(9):1061-3.

[A case of sleep apnea syndrome with significant alteration of apnea index by sleep position].
Nippon Kyobu Shikkan Gakkai Zasshi. 1993 Aug;31(8):1034-9.
Japanese.

Effect of sleep position on obstructive sleep apnea.
Tohoku J Exp Med. 1988 Dec;156 Suppl:143-9.

Sleep apnea and body position during sleep.
Sleep. 1988 Feb;11(1):90-9.

The sleep supine position has a major effect on optimal nasal continuous positive airway pressure.
Chest. 1999 Oct;116(4):1000

Positional vs nonpositional obstructive sleep apnea patients: anthropomorphic, nocturnal polysomnographic, and multiple sleep latency test data.
Chest. 1997 Sep;112(3):629-39.

The effects of posture on obstructive sleep apnea.
Am Rev Respir Dis. 1986 Apr;133(4):662-6.

Upright body position and weight loss improve respiratory mechanics and daytime oxygenation in obese patients with obstructive sleep apnoea.
Clin Physiol. 2000 Jan;20(1):50-5.

Idiopathic intracranial hypertension without papilledema: related to sleep apnea?
Arch Neurol. 1992 Jan;49(1):14.

Raised intracranial pressure syndrome of non tumourous origin in children aged up to 3 years.
Acta Univ Carol Med Monogr. 1976;(75):123-4.

Mechanisms of obstructive sleep apneas in infants.
Biol Neonate. 1994;65(3-4):235-9. Review.

Sleep position training as treatment for sleep apnea syndrome: a preliminary study.
Sleep. 1985; 8(2): 87-94.

Sleeping position and sleep apnea syndrome.
Am J Otolaryngol. 1985 Sep-Oct; 6(5): 373-7.

A comparative study of treatments for positional sleep apnea.
Tohoku J Exp Med. 1988 Jan;154(1):91-2.

Effect of sleep state and position on the incidence of obstructive and central apnea in infants.
Pediatrics. 1985 May;75(5):832-5.

SUDDEN INFANT DEATH SYNDROME and SLEEP POSITION, BRAIN PRESSURE

Here is another field, SIDS, that has looked at head position during sleep. Too bad one specialty rarely communicates with another.

Glossary:

ependymal = refers to the membrane lining of the brain ventricles
medulla = part of the brain
pons = part of the brain
prone = lying with the face downward

[Chronic intracranial pressure and SIDS]
Dtsch Med Wochenschr. 1987 Frb;112(6):239. German.

Sleeping position and SIDS.
Lancet. 1988 Jul 9;2(8602):106.

Sudden infant death syndrome related to sleeping position and bedding.
Med J Aust. 1991 Oct 21;155(8):507-8. Review.

The effect of head elevation on intracranial pressure in the neonate.
Crit Care Med. 1983 Jun;11(6):428-30

Assessment of infant sleeping position –selected states, 1996. (From the Centers for Disease Control and Prevention)
JAMA. 1998 Dec 9;280(22):1899

Sudden infant death syndrome: near-weightlessness and delayed neural transformation.
Med Hypotheses. 1996 Apr;46(4):383-7. Review.

Vertebral artery compression resulting from head movement: A possible cause of Sudden Infant Death Syndrome.
Pediatrics. 1999 Feb;103 (2):460-1

Prevalence and determinants of prone sleeping position in infants: results from two cross-sectional studies on risk factors for SIDS in Germany.
American J Epidemiology. 1999 July 1:150(1):51-7

Babies sleeping with parents: case-control study of factors influencing the risk for the sudden infant death syndrome.
Br Med J. 1999 Dec;319(7223):1457

Infant cranial molding deformation and sleep position: implications for primary care.
J Pediatr Health Care. 1999 Jul-Aug;13(4):173-7.

Skull morphology affected by different sleep positions in infancy.
Cleft Palate Craniofac J. 1995 Sep;32(5):413-9

Still need to stress back sleep for infants to parents.
Family Practice News. 1999 Nov;29(21):42

Sudden infant death syndrome: postnatal changes in the volumes of the pons, medulla, and cervical spinal cord.
J Neuropathol Exp Neurol. 1995 Jul;54(4):570-80

Brain weight and sudden infant death syndrome.
J Child Neurol. 1995 Mar;10(2):123-6

Organ weights in sudden infant death syndrome.
Pediatr Pathol. 1994 Nov-Dec;14(6):973-85

Cerebral CT in fatal courses of resuscitated sudden infant death.
AJNR Am J Neuroradiol. 1983 May-Jun;4(3):689-91

Infant apnea syndrome. A prospective evaluation of etiologies.
Clin Pediatr (Phila.) 1982 Nov;21(11):684-7

A contribution to a possible differentiation between SIDS and asphyxiation.
Forensic Sci Int. 1998 Jan 30;91(2):147-52

Ependymal changes in sudden infant death syndrome.
J Neuropathol Exp Neurol. 1996 Mar;55(3):348-56

EPILEPSY and MIGRAINE, BRAIN EDEMA

Epilepsy is related to migraines and brain edema, but the connection between these factors and sleep is not considered, as usual.

Glossary:

pleocytosis = increased white blood cells (lymphocytes) in spinal fluid
status epilepticus = a series of epileptic seizures in rapid succession

[Migraine and epilepsy].
Schweiz Rundsch Med Prax. 1982 Oct 12;71(41):1595-9. German.

Migraines and epilepsies—a relationship?
Epilepsia. 1966 Mar;7(1):53-66.

Migraine and epilepsy: a retrospective view.
Funct Neurol. 1986 Oct-Dec;1(4):559-61.

The relation of migraine and epilepsy.
Brain. 1969;92(2):285-300.

Migraine and epilepsy.
Dev Med Child Neurol. 1992 Jul;34(7):645-7. Review.

Migraine and epilepsy.
Neurol Clin. 1994 Feb;12(1):115-28. Review.

On the relationship migraine—epilepsy.
Nebr State Med J. 1971 Apr;56(4):136-9.

A case-control study to evaluate the association of epilepsy and migraine.
Neuroepidemiology. 1992;11(4-6):313-4.

Migraine and epilepsy.
Neurol Clin. 1997 Feb;15(1):107-14. Review.

Migraine and epilepsy.
Folia Psychiatr Neurol Jpn. 1980;34(3):405-6.

Migraine and epilepsy.
Eur Neurol. 1970;3(3):168-78.

[Convulsions caused by migraine].
Arch Fr Pediatr. 1979 May;36(5):498-501

Appearing and disappearing CT scan abnormalities and seizures.
J Neurol Neurosurg Psychiatry. 1985 Sep;48(9):866-9.

Prolonged focal cerebral edema associated with partial status
epilepticus.
Epilepsia. 1985 Jul-Aug;26(4):334-9.

Migraine associated with focal cerebral edema, cerebrospinal fluid
pleocytosis, and progressive cerebellar ataxia: MRI documentation.
Neurology. 1990 Aug;40(8):1284-7.

[Relations between migraine and epilepsy].
Munch Med Wochenschr. 1965 Sep 17;107(38):1843-7. German.

PARKINSON'S DISEASE and BRAIN EDEMA, BRAIN CIRCULATION

Parkinson's disease has been known to involve extra brain fluid and reduced brain circulation.

Glossary:

aqueductal stenosis = narrowing of the channels between brain ventricles, inhibiting the flow of cerebral spinal fluid
hydrocephalus = excess fluid in the brain
vertbrobasilar insufficiency = reduced blood circulation in the back of the brain

Parkinsonism and acquired hydrocephalus.
Mov Disord. 1986;1(1):59-64.

Parkinsonism associated with obstructive hydrocephalus due to idiopathic aqueductal stenosis.
J Neurol Neurosurg Psychiatry. 1998 May;64(5):657-9. Review.

Regional cerebral blood flow during an attack of vertebrobasilar insufficiency.
Stroke. 1988 Nov;19(11):1426-30.

A case of normal pressure hydrocephalus presenting as levodopa responsive parkinsonism.
J Neurol Neurosurg Psychiatry. 1987 Feb;50(2):234. No abstract available.

Parkinsonian syndromes associated with hydrocephalus: case reports, a review of the literature, and pathophysiological hypotheses.
Mov Disord. 1994 Sep;9(5):508-20. Review.

Parkinson's disease and hydrocephalus.
Adv Neurol. 1990;53:305-9. No abstract available.

Parkinsonian syndrome in the course of aqueductal stenosis hydrocephalus.
Ital J Neurol Sci. 1988 Dec;9(6):603-6.

Obstructive hydrocephalus-induced parkinsonism. I: Decreased basal ganglia regional blood flow.
Pediatr Neurol. 1988 Mar-Apr;4(2):117-9.

ORGASM AND IMPOTENCE and their relationship to MIGRAINE, SLEEP APNEA, AND STROKE

The presence of brain edema in the above diseases has been under-appreciated by researchers, who have had no clue as to the cause of the edema and therefore have ignored its implications. It is no surprise, then, that they have also under-appreciated diseases of body structures outside of the skull that may result from brain edema. It is clear, however, that impotence is an issue that involves the bed and head elevation, and is related to other brain conditions involving the same thing, such as sleep apnea, migraines, and stroke. And when you consider side and stomach sleeping and its effect on the genitals, as we discussed, it is obvious that impotence could be all in your bed.

Glossary:

cephalgia = headache
coitus = sex
penile tumescence = erections

Stroke and orgasmic cephalgia.
Headache. 1981 Jan;21(1):12-3.

[Sexual headache and cerebral hemorrhage].
Rev Neurol. 1995 Jan-Feb;23(119):184-5. Spanish.

Orgasm—a new trigger factor of cluster headache?
Cephalalgia. 1990 Aug;10(4):205-6.

When sex is a headache.
BMJ. 1991 Jul 27;303(6796):202-3.

Sexually induced headaches.
Br Med J. 1977 Jun 25;1(6077):1664.

Aging, sleep disorders, and male sexual function.
Biol Psychiatry. 1991 Jul 1;30(1):15-24.

159

Erectile dysfunction in sleep apnea and response to CPAP.
J Sex Marital Ther. 1995 Winter;21(4):239-47.

Headaches associated with orgasm.
Log. 1975 May;9(5):7, 10, 15-6.

Warning headache in aneurysmal subarachnoid hemorrhage.
Arch Neurol. 1989 Aug;46(8):839.

[Cerebral hemorrhage in migraine].
Rev Neurol (Paris). 1993;149(6-7):407-10. Review. French.

Coital cerebral hemorrhage.
Neurology. 1993 Dec;43(12):2683-5.

[Sleep apnea and erectile dysfunction].
Dtsch Med Wochenschr. 1999 May 21;124(20):631-5. Review. German.

Pituitary-gonadal function during sleep in men with erectile impotence
and normal controls.
Psychosom Med. 1984 May-Jun;46(3):239-54.

Sleep-related penile tumescence as a function of age.
Am J Psychiatry. 1975 Sep;132(9):932-7.

Benign vascular sexual headache and exertional headache:
interrelationships and long term prognosis.
J Neurol Neurosurg Psychiatry. 1991 May;54(5):417-21.

Persistent segmental cerebral artery constrictions in coital cephalgia.
J Neurol Neurosurg Psychiatry. 1990 Mar;53(3):266-7.

Sexual dysfunction in female patients with multiple sclerosis.
Int Rehabil Med. 1981;3(1):32-4.

Benign orgasmic cephalgia.
Headache. 1974 Jan;13(4):181-7.

[Study of coital orgasm in women].
Cesk Gynekol. 1984 May;49(4):257-61. Czech.

Heart rate, rate-pressure product, and oxygen uptake during four sexual activities.
Arch Intern Med. 1984 Sep;144(9):1745-8.

Neuroendocrine and cardiovascular response to sexual arousal and orgasm in men.
Psychoneuroendocrinology. 1998 May;23(4):401-11.

Migraine angiitis precipitated by sex headache and leading to watershed infarction.
Cephalalgia. 1993 Dec;13(6):427-30.

Benign orgasmic cephalgia.
Trans Am Neurol Assoc. 1973;98:295-7.

[Coitus as a factor in the pathogenesis of neurologic complications].
Cesk Neurol. 1970 May;33(3):162-7. Czech.

Masturbatory-orgasmic extracephalic pain.
Headache. 1998 Feb;38(2):138-41.

Erectile dysfunction in hypertensive subjects. Assessment of potential determinants.
Hypertension. 1996 Nov;28(5):859-62.

Hypertension and impotence.
Eur Urol. 1991;19(1):29-34.

Erectile dysfunction in diabetes and hypertension.
Urology. 1985 Aug;26(2):135-7.

Hypothalamic-hypophyseal-testicular abnormalities and erectile dysfunction.
Arch Androl. 1988;20(2):137-40.

Erectile dysfunction in hypertensive men: sleep-related erections, penile blood flow and musculovascular events.
J Urol. 1989 Jul;142(1):56-61.

Nightly variability in the indices of sleep-disordered breathing in men being evaluated for impotence with consecutive night polysomnograms.
Sleep. 1996 Sep;19(7):589-92.

Pituitary-gonadal function during sleep in men with hypoactive sexual desire and in normal controls.
Psychosom Med. 1988 May-Jun;50(3):304-18.

Sleep and sexual function in the elderly male.
Biol Psychiatry. 1991 Jul 1;30(1):1-3.

Problems in the interpretation of nocturnal penile tumescence studies: disruption of sleep by occult sleep disorders.
J Urol. 1986 Sep;136(3):595-8.

Diabetes, sleep disorders, and male sexual function.
Biol Psychiatry. 1993 Aug 1;34(3):171-7.

Hypertension, erectile dysfunction, and occult sleep apnea.
Sleep. 1989 Jun;12(3):223-32.

Prevalence of sleep apnea in men with erectile dysfunction.
Urology. 1990 Sep;36(3):232-4.

HEAD ELEVATION AND SLEEP POSITION and BRAIN PRESSURE, BRAIN CIRCULATION, AND THE TREATMENT OF BRAIN EDEMA

Researchers knew that lying flat causes brain edema. They knew that brain edema is associated with many brain conditions. The following shows that they already use head elevation to reduce brain edema in the treatment of some conditions.

Glossary:

anti-orthostatic hypokinesia = hanging upside-down
intracranial = inside the brain
perfusion pressure = the pressure for fluid to pass out of a blood vessel into the surrounding tissue

Effects of neck position on intracranial pressure.
Am J Crit Care. 1993 Jan;2(1):68-71.

Cerebral perfusion pressure, intracranial pressure, and head elevation.
J Neurosurg. 1986 Nov;65(5):636-41.

Head position affects intracranial pressure in newborn infants.
J Pediatr. 1983 Dec;103(6):950-3.

Intracranial pressure changes during positioning of patients with severe head injury.
Heart Lung. 1989 Jul;18(4):411-4.

Sleeping positions.
Pediatrics. 1992 Nov;90(5):782.

[The sleeping position and its consequences over health and the mouth].
Majallat Tibb Alfamm Alsuriyah. 1976 Mar;12(1):16-21. Arabic.

[The sleeping position and deformities caused by compression: an alert for outpatient pediatricians. Letter].
An Esp Pediatr. 1997 Mar;46(3):313-4. Spanish.

[On the dangers and problems of the horizontal position during sleeping hours].
Tidsskr Nor Laegeforen. 1965 Dec 1;85(23):1757-61. Norwegian.

Changes in cerebral blood volume with changes in position in awake and anesthetized subjects.
Anesth Analg. 2000 Feb;90(2):372-6.

Left or right, up or down: a case for positioning of unconscious head-injured patients.
Curationis. 1992 Apr;15(1):1-7.

The effects of patient repositioning on intracranial pressure.
Aust J Adv Nurs. 1994 Dec-1995 Feb;12(2):32-9.

The effect of nursing activities on intracranial pressure.
Br J Nurs. 1994 May 12-25;3(9):454-9. Review.

Trends in the care and treatment of patients with increased intracranial pressure.
Axone. 1992 Jun;13(4):125-8.

Practical points in understanding intracranial pressure.
J Post Anesth Nurs. 1994 Dec;9(6):357-9.

The effect of head position on intracranial pressure in the neonate.
Crit Care Med. 1983 Jun;11(6):428-30.

[Patient posture in neurosurgery].
Ann Fr Anesth Reanim. 1995;14(1):90-4.

Intracranial pressure: dynamics and nursing management.
J Neurosci Nurs. 1991 Apr;23(2):85-91. Review.

[The effect of position on intracranial pressure].
Ann Fr Anesth Reanim. 1998;17(2):149-56. Review. French.

Influence of body position on jugular venous oxygen saturation, intracranial pressure and cerebral perfusion pressure.
Acta Neurochir Suppl (Wien). 1993;59:107-12.

Cerebral and cardiovascular responses to changes in head elevation in patients with intracranial hypertension.
J Neurosurg. 1983 Dec;59(6):938-44.

Management of head injury. Treatment of abnormal intracranial pressure.
Neurosurg Clin N Am. 1991 Apr;2(2):267-84. Review.

Effect of backrest position on intracranial and cerebral perfusion pressures.
J Neurosci Nurs. 1990 Dec;22(6):375-81.

Influence of body position on tissue-pO2, cerebral perfusion pressure and intracranial pressure in patients with acute brain injury.
Neurol Res. 1997 Jun;19(3):249-53.

[Intracranial pressure monitoring in clinical practice. Report of 180 cases].
Chung Hua I Hsueh Tsa Chih. 1989 Feb;69(2):90-2, 8.

Intracranial pressure. Monitoring and management.
Neurosurg Clin N Am. 1994 Oct;5(4):573-605. Review.

Intracranial pressure: a review of clinical problems, measurement techniques and monitoring methods.
J Med Eng Technol. 1986 Nov-Dec;10(6):299-320. Review.

Effect of head elevation on intracranial pressure, cerebral perfusion pressure, and cerebral blood flow in head-injured patients.
J Neurosurg. 1992 Feb;76(2):207-11.

Head position, intracranial pressure, and compliance.
Neurology. 1982 Nov;32(11):1288-91.

Control of intracranial pressure in patients with severe head injury.
J Neurotrauma. 1992 Mar;9 Suppl 1:S317-26.

Positioning and intracranial hypertension: implications of the new critical pathway for nursing practice.
Off J Can Assoc Crit Care Nurs. 1998 Winter;9(4):12-6; quiz 17-8. Review.

[Treatment of increased intracranial pressure in craniocerebral trauma].
Langenbecks Arch Chir Suppl Kongressbd. 1997;114:198-202. Review.

Management of intracranial hemodynamics in the adult: a research
analysis of head positioning and recommendations for clinical practice
and future research.
J Neurosci Nurs. 1997 Feb;29(1):44-9. Review.

Intracranial Pressure/ Head Elevation.
http://pedsccm.wustl.edu/All-Net/spanish/neurpage/protect/icp-tx-
3.htm

Effect of head-down tilt on brain water distribution.
Eur J Appl Physiol. 1999 Mar;79(4):367-73.

MISCELLANEOUS

Sydney Ross Singer and Soma Grismaijer. Dressed To Kill: The Link Between Breast Cancer and Bras. Avery Pub. Group, NY. 1995

Colligan, Douglas. Creative Insomnia. Franklin Watts, NY 1978

Rodale, JI. Sleep and Rheumatism. Rodale Books, Inc. Emmaus, Penn. 1940

Turkington, Carol. The Brain Encyclopedia. Fact on File, Inc. NY 1996

Simpson, Carolyn. Coping with Sleep Disorders. The Rosen Pub. Group, Inc. NY 1996

Powledge, Tabitha M. Your Brain: How You Got It and How It Works. Charles Scribner's Sons, Inc., NY 1994

Cecil Essentials of Medicine, Second Ed. W.B. Saunders Company, Phil., Pa. 1990

Melloni's Illustrated Medical Dictionary. The Williams and Wilkens Co., Baltimore, MD 1979

As you can see, the pieces are all there. The medical research industry knows about head elevation. They are simply not talking about it.

Postscript

It has been several months since the first printing of ***Get It Up!*** We have encouraged Self Study participants to try head elevation for different conditions, in addition to the many we have already discussed in this book, and are excited to report that it has worked for asthma, attention deficit disorder, middle ear infections, and some allergies. The number of participants is too small at this time for a major announcement of results. But the results were dramatic, and everyone who tried head elevation has benefited by some form of improved health. Everyone reported less sinus congestion in the morning.

The asthma connection suggests that the brain stem and its respiratory control centers are impaired in asthma, just as they are in SIDS and sleep apnea. In fact, asthma is also associated with migraines, is worse in the morning, and is related to sleep disorders.

Attention deficit hyperactivity disorder, or ADHD, is also associated with sleep problems, asthma, migraines, and stuffy sinuses. Within a month of sleeping elevated, the kids who tried this were off of their medication and completely normal. They awoke easier, had a better attitude, performed better in school, had less congestion in the sinuses, and no longer had asthma or migraine attacks.

Children who suffered from recurrent middle ear infections found relief by sleeping on their backs, elevated. Side and stomach sleeping compresses the ear into the bed or pillow, creating a compression injury. And it is medically known that middle ear pressure, like eye pressure, goes up when the head goes down, and vice versa. So sleeping flat and compressing the ear are what cause these infections. Recovery is quick once the sleep position is corrected.

Some people who tried head elevation realized within days that they were no longer allergic to their animals. Some other people reported less eye dryness upon awakening in the morning. Many reported an end to insomnia and the best sleep they had had in years.

We also discovered that the nursing profession knows about head elevation, calling it "Fowler's position". This position is about a 30-degree elevation and is used for many conditions. Interestingly, it is also used after thyroid surgery, better allowing the throat tissue to drain. Of course, this suggests that lying flat could make thyroid tissue congested, impairing its function. Therefore, people suffering from low thyroid may benefit from head elevation to better drain their thyroid and improve its circulation.

We also came to realize that making a 10-degree full incline plane by placing blocks underneath the front legs of the bed works well, particularly for children. This may make elevation easier to try. But be aware of congestion in the feet and legs to make sure they are not getting too much fluid. This is more of a concern for anyone with leg circulation problems. Children, on the other hand, should have no trouble with this technique, and it seems to be the easiest way to get kids to sleep elevated.

We also found that many people simply propped their bodies up with pillows, and it worked. So try different techniques for elevation to see what works for you.

The success of head elevation in improving so many disease conditions is clearly related to the central role that the brain plays in the control and modification of all bodily functions. When the brain is congested and malfunctioning, anything can go wrong. This means that *every* health problem might be improved by head elevation. As our research continues, we'll keep you posted. Better yet, do the research on yourself, and keep *us* posted!

Notes

[1] Khaltaev, Nikolai "Inter-Health Fights Lifestyle Diseases" (World Health Organization; Inter-Health Program) World Health, May-Jun 1991

[2] Blau, JN. Migraine: theories of pathogenesis. Lancet 1992;339:1202-1207

[3] Discussion, ideas abound in migraine research; consensus remains elusive. JAMA. 1987 Jan 2;257(1):9-12

[4] Hargens AR Fluid shifts in vascular and extravascular spaces during and after simulated weightlessness. Med Sci Sports Exerc 1983;15(5):421-7
"Subjects were tilted 5-degrees head down for 8 h to determine vascular and extravascular shifts of fluid. Most of the initial loss of leg volume during head down tilt represented a passive shift of venous blood toward the head. Facial edema, headache, nasal congestion, and a pronounced diuresis were associated with a redistribution of blood volume."

Parazynski SE, Hargens AR, Tucker B, Aratow M, Styf J, Crenshaw A. Transcappilary fluid shifts in tissues of the head and neck during and after simulated microgravity. J Appl Physiol 1991 Dec;71(6):2469-75

Hargens AR. Recent bed rest results and countermeasure developments at NASA. Acta Physiol Scand Suppl 1994;616:103-14
"...increased capillary perfusion in tissues of the head cause facial and intracranial edema. Intracranial pressure increases from 2 to 17 mm Hg going from upright posture to 6-degrees head down tilt."

[5] Moffett AM, et al. Effect of chocolate on migraine: a double-blind study. J Neurol Neurosurg Psychiatry 1974;37:445-48

[6] Kroeglstein G; Langham ME. Influence of body position on the intraocular pressure of normal and glaucomatous eyes. Opthalmologica 1975;171(2):132-45
"In a series of six lowtension glaucomatous eyes the postural response was significant as a probable pathogenetic factor in that disease, because the intraocular pressure could rise from a normal to a glaucomatous level upon changing from the seated to the supine position."

[7] Weinreb RN; Cook J; Friberg TR. Effect of inverted position on intraocular pressure. Am J Opthalmol 1984 Dec 15;98(6):784-7
"We recommend that patients with ocular hypertension or glaucoma refrain from this activity."

[8] Williams ML. The sinusitis help book: a comprehensive guide to a common problem: questions, answers, options. Chronimed Pub., Minn., MN 1998

[9] Sleep. The Universal World Reference Encyclopedia (unabridged); Chicago, 1945

Index

ABOUT THE AUTHORS

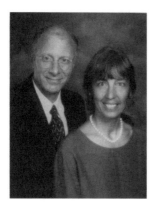 **Sydney Ross Singer** and **Soma Grismaijer** are a husband-and-wife research team dedicated to uncovering the lifestyle causes of disease. Medical anthropologists and co-authors of, *Dressed To Kill: The Link Between Breast Cancer and Bras* (Avery, 1995), *Get It Up!, Get It Off!,* and *Get It Out!,* (ISCD Press, 2000-2001) this dynamic duo is known worldwide for their willingness to stand up to the profit-oriented, treatment focused medical system.

Sydney Ross Singer received a B.S. in biology from the University of Utah in 1979. He then spent two years in the biochemistry Ph.D. program at Duke University, followed by another two years at Duke in the anthropology Ph.D. program, receiving a Master's Degree. He then attended the University of Texas Medical Branch (UTMB) at Galveston, Texas on a full academic scholarship, where he spent one year in the medical humanities Ph.D. program, and received an additional two years training in medical school.

Soma Grismaijer received an associate's degree from the College of Marin in the behavioral sciences, and a bachelor of arts from Sonoma State University in environmental studies and planning. In addition, she is an American Board of Opticianry-certified optician. She has been the President and Executive Director of the Good Shepherd Foundation since 1980, a charitable organization dedicated to the elimination of human and animal suffering.

Together, Singer and Grismaijer started the Institute for the Study of Culturogenic Disease in 1991. Their first project was the M.D. (Medical Demystification) Crusade, informing the public of the hazards of medicine and how to prevent them. The Crusade included the Medication Side Effects Hotline, and a national lecture tour explaining the nature of doctors, medicine, and health. Following their research into the cause of breast cancer and the publication of **Dressed To Kill**, Singer and Grismaijer traveled around the world bringing their health message to millions of people. Currently, they are spearheading an international campaign to educate people about various culturogenic diseases, explaining how to prevent and cure a host of conditions considered a "mystery" by modern medicine . In addition, they have begun an Internet based SELF STUDY CENTER, at selfstudycenter.org, to help people practice health self-care by trying certain lifestyle changes.

Singer and Grismaijer, and their 9 year-old Solomon, practice what they preach in Hawaii, on a 67-acre tropical rainforest preserve.